CW01024872

50 Studies Every Intensivist Should Know

50 Studies Every Doctor Should Know

50 Studies Every Intensivist Should Know

EDITED BY

EDWARD A. BITTNER, MD, PHD, MSED
Program Director, Critical Care-Anesthesiology Fellowship
Associate Director, Surgical Intensive Care Unit
Massachusetts General Hospital
Associate Professor of Anaesthesia
Harvard Medical School
Boston, MA

SERIES EDITOR:

MICHAEL E. HOCHMAN, MD, MPH
Associate Professor, Medicine
Director, Gehr Family Center for Health Systems Science
USC Keck School of Medicine
Los Angeles, CA

OXFORD
UNIVERSITY PRESS

OXFORD
UNIVERSITY PRESS

Oxford University Press is a department of the University of Oxford. It furthers
the University's objective of excellence in research, scholarship, and education
by publishing worldwide. Oxford is a registered trade mark of Oxford University
Press in the UK and certain other countries.

Published in the United States of America by Oxford University Press
198 Madison Avenue, New York, NY 10016, United States of America.

© Oxford University Press 2018

All rights reserved. No part of this publication may be reproduced, stored in
a retrieval system, or transmitted, in any form or by any means, without the
prior permission in writing of Oxford University Press, or as expressly permitted
by law, by license, or under terms agreed with the appropriate reproduction
rights organization. Inquiries concerning reproduction outside the scope of the
above should be sent to the Rights Department, Oxford University Press, at the
address above.

You must not circulate this work in any other form
and you must impose this same condition on any acquirer.

Library of Congress Cataloging-in-Publication Data
Names: Bittner, Edward A., 1967– editor.
Title: 50 studies every intensivist should know / edited by Edward A. Bittner.
Other titles: Fifty studies every intensivist should know |
50 studies every doctor should know (Series)
Description: Oxford ; New York : Oxford University Press, [2018] |
Series: 50 studies every doctor should know
Identifiers: LCCN 2017030839 | ISBN 9780190467654 (pbk. : alk. paper)
Subjects: | MESH: Critical Care | Evidence-Based Medicine | Clinical Trials as Topic
Classification: LCC R852 | NLM WX 218 | DDC 610.72/4—dc23
LC record available at https://lccn.loc.gov/2017030839

This material is not intended to be, and should not be considered, a substitute for medical or other
professional advice. Treatment for the conditions described in this material is highly dependent on the
individual circumstances. And, while this material is designed to offer accurate information with respect
to the subject matter covered and to be current as of the time it was written, research and knowledge about
medical and health issues is constantly evolving and dose schedules for medications are being revised
continually, with new side effects recognized and accounted for regularly. Readers must therefore always
check the product information and clinical procedures with the most up-to-date published product
information and data sheets provided by the manufacturers and the most recent codes of conduct and safety
regulation. The publisher and the authors make no representations or warranties to readers, express or
implied, as to the accuracy or completeness of this material. Without limiting the foregoing, the publisher
and the authors make no representations or warranties as to the accuracy or efficacy of the drug dosages
mentioned in the material. The authors and the publisher do not accept, and expressly disclaim, any
responsibility for any liability, loss or risk that may be claimed or incurred as a consequence of the use
and/or application of any of the contents of this material.

9 8 7 6 5 4 3 2 1

Printed by WebCom, Inc., Canada

CONTENTS

SECTION 8 Endocrine

SECTION 9 Musculoskeletal

PREFACE

There has been an explosion of clinical trials in critical care medicine since the inception of the specialty more than 50 years ago. This explosion has made it challenging as a trainee in critical care medicine to gain expertise in evidence based medicine. Determining how best to care for patients and understanding the basis for our practice is a never-ending process for all clinicians and it is particularly daunting for trainees. Even for the practicing intensivist, feeling confident in one's knowledge base of foundational studies in the ever-growing field of critical care practice is no easy task.

No single book can provide the knowledge acquired through years of study and clinical experience. However, the goal of this book is to provide an introduction to core clinical trials and studies in critical care that have and continue to impact practice. It is meant as a starting point allowing the learner to comfortably wade into the shallow end of the critical care knowledge pool rather than jumping in immediately at the deep end.

By design each chapter summarizes a trial or study in a format that is brief enough to be understood by a resident or new fellow entering a critical care rotation yet comprehensive enough to be relevant for a critical care attending physician. We also sought to highlight the limitations and generalizability of each study.

Importantly, some of the studies summarized in this book no longer represent the standard of care, yet they were chosen for inclusion because their impact on clinical practice has continued to shape the way in which critical care medicine is practiced. My hope is that this book will fill an unmet need for trainees, non-intensivists, and even some practicing intensivists by placing the current critical care literature in context.

The greatest challenge in putting this book together was selecting which 50 studies to include. Selection of studies that emphasize topics that come up frequently on ICU rounds was a priority. By necessity, content areas that had been studied in large clinical trials were emphasized. While the selection of studies for this book were peer reviewed by a national group of educators in critical care medicine, inevitably some key studies were left off the list; this leaves the opportunity for "another *50 Studies Every Intensivist Should Know*" in the future.

As an initial volume this book should be considered a work in progress—I welcome your feedback as to the studies that have been included or excluded, and if the book has future editions this information will be useful to refine its contents. Thank you for reading this book; I hope that you will find it useful.

Edward A. Bittner, MD, PhD, MSEd

ACKNOWLEDGMENTS

This book was only made possible by the collective efforts of our contributors: by and large fellows and faculty in the Departments of Anesthesiology, Medicine, and Surgery at the Massachusetts General Hospital. Many thanks for the hours of work that they put into writing and revising the chapters in the book.

I would like to thank Dr. Michael Hochman, the 50 Studies editor, and Oxford University Press for the opportunity to make this book a reality. I would like to also thank the anonymous peer review panel of critical care educators recruited by Oxford University Press who helped narrow down the list of studies and recommended publication of this volume.

Finally I would like to thank the following authors of the original studies summarized in this book who were kind enough to spend time reviewing its content. Importantly, however, any errors contained in this book do not represent those of the authors or reviewers acknowledged hereafter; any mistakes are my own.

Dr. Olaf Bakker, first author: Early versus on-demand nasoenteric tube feeding in acute pancreatitis. *N Engl J Med.* 2014;371(21):1983–1993.

Dr. Renaldo Bellomo, first author: Low-dose dopamine in patients with early renal dysfunction: a placebo-controlled randomized trial. *Lancet.* 2000; 356:2139–2143.

Dr. Gordon Bernard, first author: Efficacy and safety of recombinant human activated protein C for severe sepsis. *N Engl J Med.* 2001;344:699–709.

Dr. Roy Brower, first author: The acute respiratory distress syndrome network: ventilation with lower tidal volumes as compared with traditional tidal volumes for acute lung injury and the acute respiratory distress syndrome. *N Engl J Med.* 2000, 342:1301–1308.

Dr. Randall Chesnut, first author: A trial of intracranial-pressure monitoring in traumatic brain injury. *N Engl J Med.* 2012;367(26):2471–2481.

Dr. Jamie Cooper, first author: Decompressive craniectomy in diffuse traumatic brain injury. *N Engl J Med.* 2011;364(16):1493–1502.

Dr. Daniel De Backer, first author: Comparison of dopamine and norepinephrine in the treatment of shock. *N Engl J Med.* 2010;362:779–789.

Dr. Andres Esteban, first author, Spanish Lung Failure Collaborative Group: A comparison of four methods of weaning patients from mechanical ventilation. *N Engl J Med.* 1995;332(6):345–350.

Dr. Claude Guérin, first author: Prone positioning in severe acute respiratory distress syndrome. *N Engl J Med.* 2013;368(23):2159–2168.

Dr. Simon Finfer, first author: The SAFE Study Investigators: A comparison of albumin and saline for fluid resuscitation in the intensive care unit. *N Engl J Med.* 2004;350(22):2247–2256.

Dr. Paul Hébert, first author: Transfusion Requirements in Critical Care Investigators, Canadian Critical Care Trials Group: A multicenter, randomized, controlled clinical trial of transfusion requirements in critical care. *N Engl J Med.* 1999;340(6):409.

Dr. Daren Heyland, first author: A randomized trial of glutamine and antioxidants in critically ill patients. *N Engl J Med.* 2013;368(16):1489–1497.

Dr. John Holcomb, first author: Transfusion of plasma, platelets, and red blood cells in a 1:1:1 vs a 1:1:2 ratio and mortality in patients with severe trauma: The PROPPR Randomized Clinical Trial. *JAMA.* 2015;313(5):471–482.

Dr. Michael Holzer, first author: The Hypothermia after Cardiac Arrest Study Group: Mild therapeutic hypothermia to improve the neurologic outcome after cardiac arrest. *N Engl J Med.* 2002;346:549–556.

Dr. Alan E. Jones, first author: Lactate clearance vs. central venous oxygen saturation as goals of early sepsis therapy: a randomized clinical trial. *JAMA.* 2010;303(8):739–746.

Dr. John Kress, first author: Daily interruption of sedative infusions in critically ill patients undergoing mechanical ventilation. *N Engl J Med.* 2000 May 18;342(20):1471–1477.

Dr. Alain Mercat, first author: Positive end-expiratory pressure setting in adults with acute lung injury and acute respiratory distress syndrome: a randomized controlled trial. *JAMA.* 2008;299(6):646–55.

Dr. Paul Palevsky, first author, VA/NIH Acute Renal Failure Trial Network: Intensity of renal support in critically ill patients with acute kidney injury. *N Engl J Med.* Jul 3 2008;359(1):7–20.

Dr. Giles Peek, first author: Efficacy and economic assessment of conventional ventilatory support versus extracorporeal membrane oxygenation for severe adult respiratory failure (CESAR): a multicenter randomized controlled trial. *Lancet.* 2009;374(9698):1351–1363.

Dr. Peter Pronovost, first author: An intervention to decrease catheter-related bloodstream infections in the ICU. *N Engl J Med.* 2006;355(26):2725–2732.

Dr. Todd Rice, first author: Initial trophic vs full enteral feeding in patients with acute lung injury: the EDEN randomized trial. *JAMA.* 2012;307(8):795–803.

Dr. Emanuel Rivers, first author, Early Goal-Directed Therapy Collaborative Group: Early goal directed therapy in the treatment of severe sepsis and septic shock. *N Engl J Med.* 2001;345(19):1368–1377.

Dr. Patrique Segers, first author: Prevention of nosocomial infection in cardiac surgery by decontamination of the nasopharynx and oropharynx with chlorhexidine gluconate: A randomized controlled trial. *JAMA.* 2006;296:2460–2466.

Dr. Charles Sprung, first author: Hydrocortisone therapy for patients with septic shock. *N Engl J Med.* 2008;358:111–124.

Dr. Thomas Strøm, first author: A protocol of no sedation for critically ill patients receiving mechanical ventilation: a randomized trial. *Lancet.* 2010 Feb 6;375(9713):475–480.

Dr. Mark S. Slaughter, first author: Advanced heart failure treated with continuous-flow left ventricular assist device. *N Engl J Med.* 2009; 361(23):2241–2251.

Dr. Daniel Talmor, first author: Mechanical ventilation guided by esophageal pressure in acute lung injury. *N Engl J Med.* 2008 Nov 13;359(20):2095–2104.

Dr. Holger Thiele, first author: Intraaortic balloon support for myocardial infarction with cardiogenic shock. *N Engl J Med.* 2012;367(14):1287–1296.

CONTRIBUTORS

Haitham S. Al Ashry, MBBCh
Fellow, Division of Pulmonary,
    Critical Care, Allergy & Sleep
    Medicine
Medical University of South Carolina
Charleston, SC

Ednan Bajwa, MD
Director, Medical Intensive Care Unit
Massachusetts General Hospital
Boston, MA

Yuriy Bronshteyn , MD
Assistant Professor, Anesthesiology
Duke University School of Medicine
Durham, NC

Kathryn Butler, MD
Instructor in Surgery
Massachusetts General Hospital
Boston, MA

Miguel Cobas, MD
Professor of Clinical Anesthesiology
Program Director, Critical Care
    Medicine Fellowship
University of Miami
Miami, FL

Andrea Coppadoro, MD
Department of Emergency and
    Urgency
A. Monzoni Hospital
Lecco, Italy

Alice Gallo De Moraes, MD
Assistant Professor of Medicine
Mayo Clinic
Rochester, MN

Marc de Moya, MD
Associate Professor and Chief,
    Division of Trauma and
    Acute Care Surgery
Medical College of Wisconsin
Milwaukee, WI

**Jose L. Diaz-Gomez , MD,
FCCM, FASE**
Chair, Department of Critical Care
    Medicine
Assistant Professor of Anesthesiology
Mayo Clinic College of Medicine
Consultant, Departments of Critical
    Care Medicine, Anesthesiology,
    and Neurosurgery
Mayo Clinic
Jacksonville, FL

David M. Dudzinski, MD
Instructor in Medicine
Massachusetts General Hospital
Boston, MA

Eric Ehieli, MD
Assistant Professor, Anesthesiology
Duke University School of Medicine
Durham, NC

Matthias Eikermann, MD, PhD
Associate Professor of Anesthesia
Massachusetts General Hospital
Boston, MA

Peter J. Fagenholz, MD
Associate Program Director, MGH
    General Surgery Residency
Massachusetts General Hospital
Boston, MA

Karim Fikry, MD
Department of Anesthesia, Critical
    Care, and Pain Medicine
Massachusetts General Hospital
Boston, MA

Guiseppe Foti, MD
Department of Emergency and
    Intensive Care
San Gerardo Hospital
School of Medicine and Surgery
University of Milan-Bicocca
Monza, Italy

Ross Gaudet, MD
Anesthesiology Fellow
Massachusetts General Hospital
Boston, MA

**Steven Greenberg, MD,
FCCP, FCCM**
Director of Critical Care Services,
    Evanston Hospital
NorthShore University HealthSystem
Clinical Associate Professor,
    Department of Anesthesiology
University of Chicago Pritzker School
    of Medicine
Chicago, IL

Melissa Grillo, MD
Assistant Professor of Clinical
    Anesthesiology
University of Miami
Miami, FL

Vadim Gudzenko, MD
Assistant Clinical Professor,
    Critical Care
Director, Critical Care Medicine
    Fellowship Program
Medical Director, PACU
Medical Director, Perioperative ICU
University of California, Los Angeles
David Geffen School of Medicine
Los Angeles, CA

Joseph R. Guenzer, MD
Assistant Professor, Anesthesiology
University of Utah Health
Salt Lake City, UT

James Sawalla Guseh, MD
Research Fellow in Medicine
Massachusetts General Hospital
Boston, MA

J. Michael Guthrie, MD
Anesthesiology Critical Care
    Medicine Fellow
University of California, Los Angeles
David Geffen School of Medicine
Los Angeles, CA

Ryan J. Horvath, MD, PhD
Staff Anesthesiologist
Massachusetts General Hospital
Boston, MA

Joseph Hyder, MD, PhD
Anesthesiologist
Mayo Clinic
Rochester, MN

Craig S. Jabaley, MD
Chief of Critical Care Medicine
Medical Director, Surgical ICU
    Anesthesiology Service Line
Atlanta VAMC
Assistant Professor of Anesthesiology
Emory University School of Medicine
South Atlanta, GA

Laleh Jalilian, MD
Clinical Instructor, Department of
    Anesthesiology
University of California, Los Angeles
David Geffen School of Medicine
Los Angeles, CA

**Namita Jayaprakash, MB, BcH,
BAO, MCEM**
Department of Pulmonary and
    Critical Care Medicine
Mayo Clinic
Rochester, MN

Christina Anne Jelly, MD, MS
Anesthesiology Resident
Massachusetts General Hospital
Boston, MA

Daniel W. Johnson, MD
Division Chief, Critical Care
Director, Critical Care Anesthesiology
    Fellowship
Associate Director,
    Cardiovascular ICU
Assistant Professor, Department of
    Anesthesiology
University of Nebraska
    Medical Center
Omaha, NE

**Haytham M. A. Kaafarani,
MD, MPH**
Director, Patient Safety & Quality,
    Trauma & Emergency Surgery
Assistant Professor of Surgery
Harvard Medical School
Boston, MA

Rebecca Kalman, MD
Anesthesiologist
Massachusetts General Hospital
Boston, MA

Jeffrey Katz, MD
Attending Anesthesiologist
NorthShore University Health
    Systems
Clinical Assistant Professor
    Department of Anesthesiology
University of Chicago Pritzker School
    of Medicine
Chicago, IL

David C. Kaufman, MD, FCCM
Professor of Surgery, Anesthesia,
  Medicine, Urology, and Medical
  Humanities and Bioethics
University of Rochester
  Medical Center
Rochester, NY

David R. King, MD, FACS
Assistant Professor of Surgery
Harvard Medical School
Director, Trauma Research Program
Associate Director, Trauma &
  Emergency Surgery Fellowship
  Program
Division of Trauma, Emergency
  Surgery, and Surgical Critical Care
Massachusetts General Hospital
Boston, MA

Jeanine Wiener Kronish, MD
Anesthetist-in-Chief
Department of Anesthesia, Critical
  Care and Pain Medicine
Massachusetts General Hospital
Boston, MA

**Avinash B. Kumar, MD,
FCCM, FCCP**
Associate Professor, Anesthesia &
  Critical Care
Medical Director, Neuro ICU
Associate Fellowship Director,
  Critical Care Fellowship
Vanderbilt University Medical Center
Nashville, TN

Jean Kwo, MD
Medical Director, Preadmission
  Testing
Department of Anesthesia, Critical
  Care & Pain Medicine
Massachusetts General Hospital
Boston, MA

Jarone Lee, MD, MPH
Medical Director, Blake 12 Surgical
  Intensive Care Unit
Quality Director, Surgical Critical
  Care, Department of Surgery
Massachusetts General Hospital
Boston, MA

Sean Levy, MD
Instructor in Medicine
Beth Israel Deaconess Medical Center
Boston, MA

Robert Loflin, MD
Critical Care Fellow
University of Rochester
  Medical Center
Rochester, NY

Laurie O. Mark, MD
Assistant Professor, Department of
  Anesthesiology
Rush University Medical College
Chicago, IL

Courtney Maxey-Jones, MD
Critical Care Fellow
University of Cincinnati Academic
  Health Center
Cincinnati, OH

Duncan McLean, MB, ChB
Anesthesiology Resident
University of Rochester
  Medical Center
Rochester, NY

Zeb McMillan, MD
Critical Care Faculty
University of California, San Diego
  School of Medicine
San Diego, CA

Angela Meier, MD, PhD
Anesthesiologist
University of California, San Diego
  Health
San Diego, CA

Pedro Mendez-Tellez, MD, PhD
Medical Director, Respiratory Care
  Services
Assistant Professor, Anesthesiology
  and Critical Care Medicine
John Hopkins Medicine
Baltimore, MD

Merrick E. Miles, MD
Assistant Professor of Anesthesiology
Division of Critical Care Medicine
Vanderbilt University Medical Center
Nashville, TN

Vivek Moitra, MD
Associate Professor, Anesthesiology
Chief, Division of Critical Care
Department of Anesthesiology
Medical Director, Cardiothoracic and
  Surgical Intensive Care Units
Program Director, Critical Care
  Medicine Fellowship program
Columbia University Medical Center
New York, NY

**Daniel J. Niven BSc, MD, MSc,
PhD, FRCPC**
Assistant Professor
Departments of Critical Care
  Medicine; Community Health
  Sciences
University of Calgary
Calgary, Canada

Ala Nozari, MD, PhD
Division Chief of Orthopedic
  Anesthesia
Associate Professor of Anaesthesia
Harvard Medical School
Boston, MA

Ameeka Pannu, MD
Clinical Fellow in Anaesthesia
Beth Israel Deaconess Medical Center
Boston, MA

Thomas Peponis, MD
Research Fellow in Surgery
Massachusetts General Hospital
Boston, MA

Richard M. Pino, MD, PhD, FCCM
Department of Anesthesia, Critical
  Care and Pain Medicine
Massachusetts General Hospital
Harvard Medical School
Boston, MA

Kimberly Pollock, MD
Assistant Clinical Professor,
  Department of Anesthesiology
University of California, San Diego
San Diego, CA

Samad Rasul, MD, FACP
Critical Care Medicine
Buffalo General Medical Center
Buffalo, NY
Olean General Hospital
Olean, NY

Sarah W. Robison, MD
Chief medical resident
Mayo Clinic
Jacksonville, FL

Daniel Saddawi-Konefka, MD
Anesthesia Residency Program
    Director
Massachusetts General Hospital
Assistant Professor, Anesthesiology
Harvard Medical School
Boston, MA

Jason L. Sanders, MD, PhD
Clinical Fellow in Medicine
Massachusetts General Hospital
Boston, MA

Dante Schiavo, MD
Internist, Pulmonologist, Critical
    Care Specialist
Mayo Clinic
Rochester, MN

Ulrich Schmidt, MD
Clinical Professor, Anesthesiology
University of California, San Diego
San Diego, CA

J. Aaron Scott, DO
Anesthesiologist/Intensivist
University of Massachusetts Memorial
    Medical Center
Worcester, MA

Shahzad Shaefi, MD
Assistant Professor of Anaesthesia
Beth Israel Deaconess Medical Center
Boston, MA

Milad Sharifpour, MD, MS
Anesthesiologist/Intensivist
Emory University School of Medicine
Atlanta, GA

Archit Sharma, MD
Anesthesiologist
University of Iowa Health Care
Iowa City, IA

Tao Shen, MD
Anesthesiologist
Massachusetts General Hospital
Boston, MA

Matthew Sigakis, MD
Clinical Lecturer, Anesthesiology
University of Michigan
    Medical School
Ann Arbor, MI

Bryan Simmons, MD
Resident in Anesthesia
Department of Anesthesia, Critical
    Care, and Pain Medicine
Massachusetts General Hospital
Boston, MA

David Stahl, MD
Department of Anesthesiology
Ohio State University Wexner
    Medical Center
Columbus, OH

Henry T. Stelfox, BMSc, MD, PhD, FRCPC
Associate Professor, Critical
   Care Medicine, Medicine and
   Community Health Sciences
University of Calgary
Calgary, Canada
Scientific Director, Alberta Health
   Services' Critical Care Strategic
   Clinical Network
Edmonton, Canada

Christopher "Kit" Tainter, MD
Assistant Professor, Departments
   of Emergency Medicine and
   Anesthesia Critical Care
University of California, San Diego
   Medical Center
San Diego, CA

Andrew Vardanian, MD
Plastic Surgeon
Resnick Neuropsychiatric Hospital
   University of California,
   Los Angeles
Los Angeles, CA

Connie Wang, MD
Resident Physician
Department of Medicine
University of California, San
   Francisco School of Medicine
San Francisco, CA

Anna M. Ward, MD
Department of Anesthesia, Critical
   Care and Pain Medicine
Massachusetts General Hospital
Harvard Medical School
Boston, MA

Gabriel Wardi, MD
Fellow, Division of Pulmonary,
   Critical Care & Sleep Medicine
University of California, San Diego
   School of Medicine
San Diego, CA

Susan R. Wilcox, MD
Associate Professor
Medical University of South
   Carolina
Charleston, SC

Michael Wolfe, MD
Critical Care and Pain Medicine
   Resident
Department of Anesthesia
Massachusetts General Hospital
Boston, MA

D. Dante Yeh, MD, FACS
Associate Professor of Surgery
Division of Trauma and Surgical
   Critical Care
The DeWitt Daughtry Family
   Department of Surgery
Ryder Trauma Center/Jackson
   Memorial Hospital
Miller School of Medicine
University of Miami
Miami, FL

50 Studies Every Intensivist Should Know

Neurologic, Sedation, and Analgesia

1

Mild Therapeutic Hypothermia to Improve the Neurologic Outcome after Cardiac Arrest

The HACA Trial

ALA NOZARI

> "In patients who have been successfully resuscitated after cardiac arrest due to ventricular fibrillation, therapeutic mild hypothermia increased the rate of a favorable neurologic outcome and reduced mortality."
>
> —THE HACA STUDY GROUP

Research Question: Does mild therapeutic hypothermia improve neurologic outcomes compared with standard care normothermia in patients surviving ventricular fibrillation or pulseless ventricular tachycardic arrest?[1]

Funding: The Biomedicine and Health Programme (BIOMED 2) of the European Union, the Austrian Ministry of Science and Transport, and the Austrian Science Foundation. Technical support and the TheraKool cooling device were provided by the Kinetic Concepts, Wareham, England.

Year Study Began: 1996

Year Study Published: 2002

Study Location: 9 centers in Austria, Belgium, Finland, Germany, and Italy.

Who Was Studied: Patients aged 18–75 years seen in the emergency department with restoration of spontaneous circulation (ROSC) after a witnessed cardiac arrest, a presumed cardiac origin of the arrest, ventricular fibrillation or non-perfusing ventricular tachycardia as the initial cardiac rhythm, an estimated interval of 5 to 15 minutes from the patient's collapse to the first resuscitation attempt by the emergency medical personnel, and an interval of ≤ 60 minutes from collapse to ROSC.

Who Was Excluded: Pregnancy, preexisting coagulopathy, temperature <30°C on admission, pre-arrest terminal illness or coma, response to verbal commands after ROSC and before randomization, cardiac arrest after arrival of emergency medical personnel, mean arterial pressure < 60 mm Hg for > 30 minutes after ROSC and before randomization, arterial oxygen saturation < 85% for > 15 minutes after ROSC, a comatose state before the cardiac arrest due to the administration of drugs, enrollment in another study, and factors that made participation in follow-up unlikely.

How Many Patients: 275

Study Overview: See Figure 1.1 for an overview of the study's design.

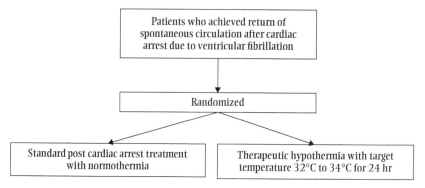

Figure 1.1 Summary of HACA's Design.

Study Intervention: All patients received standard post-cardiac arrest intensive care, including mechanical ventilation, analgesia, and sedation with fentanyl and midazolam, and neuromuscular blockade with pancuronium to prevent shivering. Normothermia was maintained in the "normothermic group" throughout the study, whereas the "hypothermia group" was cooled with an external cooling device (TheraKool, Kinetic Concepts, Wareham, England) to a target temperature of 32°C to 34°C within 4 hours after ROSC. If this goal was not achieved, additional ice packs were applied. Temperature was maintained for 24 hours, after which time passive rewarming to normothermia was allowed.

Follow-Up: Six months after arrest

Endpoints: Primary outcome was a favorable neurologic outcome, defined as the Pittsburgh Cerebral Performance Category of 1 (good recovery) or 2 (moderate disability) within 6 months after cardiac arrest. Secondary endpoints were the incidence of complications within 7 days, and mortality at 6 months.

RESULTS

- 55% of hypothermia patients had favorable neurologic outcome at 6 months, as compared to 39% in the normothermia group, yielding a relative risk (RR) of 1.40 (95% confidence interval [CI]: 1.08–1.81).
- The 6-month mortality rate was 14% lower in the normothermia group, with an RR of 0.74 (95% CI: 0.58–0.95).
- There was no group difference in the proportion of patients with complications (Table 1.1).

Table 1.1. SUMMARY OF HACA's KEY FINDINGS

Outcome	Normothermia no/total no (%)	Hypothermia	Risk Ratio	P Value
Favorable neurologic outcome	54/137 (39)	75/136 (55)	1.40 (1.08–1.81)	0.009
Death	76/138 (55)	56/137 (41)	0.74 (0.58–0.95)	0.02

Criticisms and Limitations:

- Clinicians could not be blinded to treatment assignments, which could have resulted in bias
- Only a highly selected subgroup of patients with cardiac arrest was enrolled, that is, those patients who had had a witnessed cardiac arrest and ventricular fibrillation as the initial cardiac rhythm. Previous studies suggest that less than 20% of all patients with out-of-hospital cardiac arrest belong to these subgroups.[2] Therefore, it is uncertain whether other subgroups with cardiac arrest would benefit from therapeutic hypothermia.
- The study did not evaluate the severity of coma (Glasgow Coma Scale) before randomization. Without these data, there is no reassurance that the hypothermia and normothermia groups were well matched according to the severity of the neurologic insult.

- Despite randomization, there were baseline differences in the rate of coronary artery disease and diabetes mellitus between the groups (with higher rate in the normothermia group), which might favor outcomes in the hypothermia group. However, the group difference in survival and neurological outcome remained significant despite multivariate logistic regression analysis to control for these baseline differences.
- The applied cooling technique was slow and inefficient, yielding the target temperature of 32–34°C in only 113 of 132 hypothermia patients, and not until 8 hours after ROSC. It is hence unclear whether earlier and more efficient cooling might further improve the outcome.
- It is also unclear whether therapeutic hypothermia for > 24 hours or a slower or controlled rewarming may affect the survival rate or neurological outcome in this setting. Moreover, there is no comparison between different target temperatures, and it is hence unclear whether moderate hypothermia (< 32°C) may be more effective than mild hypothermia (32–34°C).

Other Relevant Studies and Information:

- An Australian randomized controlled trial of 77 patients who had suffered cardiac arrest from ventricular fibrillation with ROSC reported improved outcomes with therapeutic hypothermia (33C for 12 h).[3]
- A recent Cochrane review concluded that mild therapeutic hypothermia improves neurological outcome after cardiac arrest, compared with no temperature management. This is consistent with current best medical practice as recommended by international resuscitation guidelines for hypothermia/targeted temperature management among survivors of cardiac arrest. However, there was insufficient evidence to show the effects of therapeutic hypothermia on participants with in-hospital cardiac arrest, asystole, or non-cardiac causes of arrest.[4]
- The Target Temperature Management after Cardiac Arrest (TTM trial) compared outcomes of 939 out-of-hospital cardiac arrest victims after cooling to 33°C versus controlled temperature maintenance at 36°C (preventing the known deleterious effect of hyperthermia).[5] The inclusion criteria included patients with out-of-hospital cardiac arrest with presenting rhythm either as ventricular fibrillation/pulseless ventricular tachycardia (VF/VT) or asystole. This rather pragmatic trial found no difference in outcome between the temperature

groups. Although the TTM study did not show additional benefits from hypothermia to 33°C as compared to 36°C, the mortality in both groups was lower than that in the control group of the HACA trial, thus suggesting the importance of active temperature management and avoidance of hyperthermia after resuscitation from cardiac arrest.

• The 2015 ACLS Guidelines recommend that comatose adult patients with ROSC after cardiac arrest (both for VF and asystole) receive TTM maintaining temperature between 32°C and 36°C for at least 24 hours after achieving target temperature.[6]

Summary and Implications: The preponderance of data suggests that temperature is an important variable for neurologic recovery after cardiac arrest. The HACA trial showed that mild therapeutic hypothermia (32–34°C) improved neurologic outcomes and reduced mortality among patients with return of spontaneous circulation after out-of-hospital cardiac arrest due to VF or pulseless VT. Recent guidelines recommend targeted temperature management for adults with cardiac arrest with either an initial shockable or nonshockable rhythm based on recent clinical trial data. Guidelines suggest maintaining a target temperature between 32°C and 36°C for at least 24 hours after achieving target temperature.

CLINICAL CASE: HYPOTHERMIA AFTER CARDIAC ARREST

Case History:
A 69-year-old man with diabetes mellitus and a history of coronary artery disease is successfully resuscitated from a ventricular fibrillation cardiac arrest, with return of spontaneous circulation. He is comatose upon arrival to the emergency department. Based on the results of HACA trial, how should this patient be treated?

Suggested Answer:
HACA trial showed that mild therapeutic hypothermia improves survival and neurological outcome in comatose survivors of ventricular fibrillation cardiac arrest. The patient in this vignette is typical of patients included in HACA. Thus, he should be cooled to 32–34°C for 24 hours after ROSC, with standard ICU care as well as therapeutic management of the hypothermia-induced shivering and other physiological effects. Although hypothermia may not be indicated for > 24 hours, the patient's temperature should be monitored to avoid hyperthermia beyond this period of treatment.

References

1. The Hypothermia after Cardiac Arrest Study Group (HACA Group). Mild therapeutic hypothermia to improve the neurologic outcome after cardiac arrest. *N Engl J Med* 2002; 346:549–556.
2. Padosch SA, Kern KB, Böttiger BW. Therapeutic hypothermia after cardiac arrest. *N Engl J Med.* 2002;347(1):63–65.
3. Bernard SA, et al. Treatment of comatose survivors of out-of-hospital cardiac arrest with induced hypothermia. *N Engl J Med* 2002;346:557–563.
4. Arrich J, Holzer M, Havel C, Müllner M, Herkner H. Hypothermia for neuroprotection in adults after cardiopulmonary resuscitation. *Cochrane Database Syst Rev.* 2016;2:CD004128.
5. Nielsen N, Wetterslev J, Cronberg T, et al. Targeted temperature management at 33°C versus 36°C after cardiac arrest. *N Engl J Med.* 2013;369(23):2197–2206.
6. Link MS, Berkow LC, Kudenchuk PJ, et al. Part 7: Adult advanced cardiovascular life support: 2015 American Heart Association Guidelines update for cardiopulmonary resuscitation and emergency cardiovascular care. *Circulation.* 2015;132(18 Suppl 2): S444–464.

2

Decompressive Craniectomy in Diffuse Traumatic Brain Injury

The DECRA Trial

MERRICK E. MILES AND AVINASH B. KUMAR

"Among adults with severe diffuse traumatic brain injury and refractory intracranial hypertension in the ICU, we found that decompressive craniectomy decreased intracranial pressure, the duration of mechanical ventilation, and the time in the ICU, as compared with standard care . . ."

—COOPER ET AL.

Research Question: Does decompressive craniectomy improve functional outcome in patients with severe traumatic brain injury (TBI) with elevated intracranial pressures (ICP) unresponsive to medical therapies?[1]

Sponsor: National Health and Medical Research Council of Australia and others

Year Study Began: 2002

Year Study Published: 2010

Study Location: 15 tertiary care hospitals in New Zealand, Australia, and Saudi Arabia

Who Was Studied: Patients 15 to 59 years old who sustained severe nonpenetrating head trauma and who did not have mass lesions. This severe trauma was defined as a Glasgow Coma Scale (GCS) of 3 to 8, or Marshall Class III (moderate to diffuse injury on computed tomography).

Who Was Excluded: Patients with mass lesions requiring surgery, patients who had spinal cord injuries, fixed and dilated pupils, or sustained cardiac arrest before arriving at the hospital. Patients who were deemed unsuitable for treatment by the clinical staff were also excluded.

How Many Patients: 155 patients were enrolled.

Study Overview: See Figure 2.1 for an overview of the study's design.

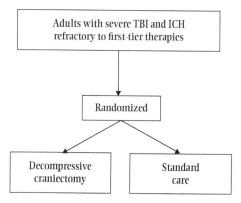

Figure 2.1 Summary of DECRA's Design.

Study Intervention: Patients with severe TBI were randomized into either a medical management group (mannitol, hypertonic saline, neuromuscular blockade, sedation, normalization of arterial carbon dioxide, and external ventricular drainage) or the medical management plus decompressive craniotomy group. If patients in the craniotomy group had ICP greater than 20 mm Hg despite medical interventions, they proceeded to decompressive craniotomy using a modified Polin technique. This technique involves bifrontal craniectomies.[2] The bone flaps were stored according to protocol and replaced in 2 to 3 months once swelling had resolved.

All patients received standard of care according to the Brain Trauma Foundation, and those randomized to medical management were allowed life-saving decompressive craniectomies after 72 hours.

Follow-Up: 36 hours after randomization and 6 months after injury

Endpoints: The original primary outcome was the proportion of patients with an unfavorable outcome, a composite of death, a vegetative state, or severe disability (a score of 1 to 4 on the Extended Glasgow Outcome Scale (GOS), although after interim analysis this was revised to be the functional outcome at 6 months after injury. Secondary outcomes were hourly ICP, the intracranial hypertension index (number of hourly ICP measurements greater than 20 mm Hg divided by total number of measurements, multiplied by 100), proportion of patients that were severely disable (defined as 2 to 4 on the Extended GOS), ICU days, hospital days and mortality.

RESULTS

- Patients in the craniectomy group, as compared with those in the medical therapy–only group, had less time with intracranial pressures above the treatment threshold ($P < 0.001$). See Table 2.1.

Table 2.1. ICP MEASUREMENT COMPARISONS BETWEEN GROUPS

Hours Since Randomization	Craniectomy Group ICP (mm Hg)	Standard of Care Group ICP (mm Hg)
–6	22	21
0	23	23
6	13	19
12	14	17
18	15	18
24	13	18

*ICP approximate

- Patients in the craniectomy group had a shorter duration of mechanical ventilation and a shorter stay in the ICU than patients in the medical therapy–only group, although there was no significant difference in total hospital length of stay.
- Hydrocephalus was more common in those patients that had undergone craniectomy (10% vs. 1%), as were complications associated with the surgery (37% vs. 17%).
- At 6-month follow-up, 70% of patients in the craniectomy group had an unfavorable outcome (functional assessment on Extended GOS) versus 51% of patients in the medical therapy–only group (odds ratio 2.21; $P < 0.02$) However, after post hoc adjustment for pupil reactivity at baseline, the differences between groups were no longer statistically significant. The outcomes evaluated by the GOS from the study are illustrated in See Table 2.2.

Table 2.2. KEY FINDINGS FROM THE DECRA TRIAL

	Craniectomy Group	Standard of Care Group	P Value
Median GOSE score[a,c]	3	4	0.03
Unfavorable outcomes[b,c]	70%	51%	0.02
Deaths	14 (19%)	15 (18%)	

[a] Extended Glasgow Outcome Scale.
[b] Defined as death, persistent vegetative state, or severe disability.
[c] Data before adjustment for pupil reactivity at baseline.

Criticisms and Limitations:

- The study had a long accrual time over which major differences in treatment may have evolved. In addition, less than 5% of screened patients were included in the trial which raises questions regarding the representativeness of the study patients.
- Normalization of ICP does not mean that brain perfusion has been improved. Measurements of cerebral blood flow, which were not performed in the study, are necessary to properly assess the value of aggressive approaches such as decompressive craniectomy in patients with traumatic brain injury.
- Eighteen percent of patients in the standard-care group had the decompressive craniectomy procedure. The impact of this crossover on the study's results is unclear.
- More patients in the decompressive craniectomy group had bilateral nonreactive pupils, radiologic findings as determined by the Marshall grading were more severe, and the GCS scale was lower compared with patients in the standard care group. These differences might suggest that the decompressive craniectomy group included a higher proportion of patients with brainstem compression or more severe injury.
- Elevated ICP was defined in the trial as > 20 mm Hg for more than 15 minutes within a 1-hour period in the study, but this maybe too low a threshold for surgical intervention or even as a valid endpoint for failure of first-tier medical management.
- The surgical technique of bifrontal craniectomy without division of the sagittal sinus and falx cerebri has been criticized as potentially an inadequate decompression, but it was chosen to decrease morbidity. Since ICP was well controlled, use of this technique was unlikely to have influenced the findings.

- The DECRA trial evaluated clinical outcomes at 6 months post injury, a practical endpoint for research. However, delayed neurologic recovery is very common following decompressive craniectomy after severe TBI with a potential for significant change up to 18 months or more.[2]
- A standardized rehabilitation process was not part of the protocol in the management of the patients enrolled in the trial.

Other Relevant Studies and Information:

- The value of decompressive craniectomy has been demonstrated in at least three randomized clinical trials for acute ischemic strokes with swelling (DECIMAL, DESTINY and HAMLET trials).[3]
- The recent multicenter RESCUEicp (Randomized Evaluation of Surgery with Craniectomy for Uncontrollable Elevation of Intracranial Pressure) trial randomly assigned 408 patients with traumatic brain injury and refractory elevated intracranial pressure (> 25 mm Hg) to undergo decompressive craniectomy or receive ongoing medical care. At 6 months, patients that had received decompressive craniectomies had lower rates of mortality and severe disability and higher rates of vegetative states than patients that received medical care alone.[4]
- Decompressive craniectomy is now most often performed for clinical and radiographic evidence of herniation, rather than for refractory ICP elevation. Consequently, results of trials that target elevated ICP alone may not directly apply to a large proportion of patients undergoing decompressive craniectomy in practice.[5]
- Studies have documented a high incidence of complications following decompressive craniectomy, including herniation of the brain outside the skull bone defects, subdural effusion, and hydrocephalus requiring ventriculo-peritoneal shunt. It may be that more attention must be directed to the prevention or optimal management of some of these complications in order to ensure that any benefit obtained by ICP management is not offset by surgical morbidity.[6]
- Guidelines from the Brain Trauma Foundation do not recommend bifrontal decompressive craniectomy for patients with severe TBI and diffuse injury (without mass lesions) and with ICP elevation that is refractory to first-tier therapies.[7]

Summary and Implications: The DECRA study established that in the context of a transient and mild increase in ICP (20 mm Hg for 15 minutes as recruitment criterion), early bifrontal decompressive craniectomy does not provide clinical benefit.

CLINICAL CASE: MANAGEMENT OF DIFFUSE TRAUMATIC BRAIN INJURY

Case History:

A 25-year-old man is admitted to the neurosciences ICU with severe diffuse traumatic brain injury following an unhelmeted high-speed motorcycle accident. On ICU day 2 his clinical examination worsens and the ICP's are more consistently in the 20 mm Hg range. Based on the results of the DECRA trial, can you make a case for urgent decompressive craniectomy?

Suggested Answer:

The DECRA study failed to demonstrate a clinical benefit early bifrontal decompressive craniectomy for patients with traumatic brain injury in the context of an ICP greater than 20 mm Hg and refractory to medical measures. At present the patient's ICPs are only mildly elevated and therefore there is no indication for surgical intervention. It is important to ensure that this patient is receiving the best available medical therapy—including adequate sedation, maintenance of a normal carbon dioxide level, optimization of blood pressure, use of osmotherapy, and drainage of cerebrospinal fluid—in a standardized, escalated manner. If ICP progresses and becomes refractory to medical treatment, decompressive craniotomy should be reconsidered.

References

1. Cooper DJ, Rosenfeld JV, Murray L, et al. Decompressive craniectomy in diffuse traumatic brain injury. *N Engl J Med.* 2011;364(16):1493–1502.
2. Ho KM, Honeybul S, Litton E. Delayed neurological recovery after decompressive craniectomy for severe nonpenetrating traumatic brain injury. *Crit Care Med.* 2011;39(11):2495–2500.
3. Vahedi K, Hofmeijer J, Juettler E, et al. Early decompressive surgery in malignant infarction of the middle cerebral artery: a pooled analysis of three randomised controlled trials. *Lancet Neurol.* 2007;6(3):215–222.
4. Hutchinson PJ, Kolias AG, Timofeev IS, et al. Trial of decompressive craniectomy for traumatic intracranial hypertension. *N Engl J Med.* 2016;375(12):1119–1130.
5. Kramer AH, Deis N, Ruddell S, et al. Decompressive craniectomy in patients with traumatic brain injury: Are the usual indications congruent with those evaluated in clinical trials? *Neurocrit Care.* 2016;25(1):10–19.
6. Honeybul S, Ho KM. Decompressive craniectomy for severe traumatic brain injury: the relationship between surgical complications and the prediction of an unfavourable outcome. *Injury.* 2014;45(9):1332–1339.
7. Brain Trauma Foundation. Guidelines for the Management of Severe Traumatic Brain Injury 4th Edition. https://braintrauma.org/uploads/03/12/ Guidelines_for_Management_of_Severe_TBI_4th_Edition.pdf. Last Accessed 4/2/2017.

3

Daily Interruption of Sedative Infusions in Critically Ill Patients Undergoing Mechanical Ventilation

DAVID STAHL

"In patients who are receiving mechanical ventilation, daily interruption of sedative drug infusions decreases the duration of mechanical ventilation and the length of stay in the intensive care unit."

—KRESS ET AL.

Research Question: Do daily interruptions of sedative and opioid infusions in critically ill patients decrease the duration of mechanical ventilation and the length of stay in the intensive care unit or hospital?[1]

Funding: None.

Year Study Began: Not explicitly stated.

Year Study Published: 2000

Study Location: Medical ICU at the University of Chicago

Who Was Studied: Critically ill patients receiving mechanical ventilation and also requiring sedation by continuous infusion.

Who Was Excluded: Patients who were admitted following cardiac arrest, transferred from another hospital where sedatives had already been administered, or those who were pregnant. Patients were also excluded if they were extubated or died within 48 hours of enrollment.

How Many Patients: 128

Study Overview: See Figure 3.1 for an overview of the study's design.

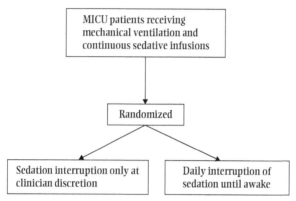

Figure 3.1 Summary of the study design.

Study Intervention: Forty-eight hours after enrollment, patients in the intervention group had their sedative and opiate infusions (either midazolam or propofol and morphine) interrupted by a research investigator until they were awake and could follow instructions, or until they became uncomfortable or agitated. Patients were deemed to be awake if they could complete 3 of 4 tasks to command: open eyes to voice, use eyes to follow the investigator on request, squeeze hand on request, stick out tongue on request. Subsequently the sedative infusions were resumed at half the previous rates, if necessary, and were adjusted to achieve a target Ramsay sedation scale of 3 or 4. Intervention patients receiving paralytic drugs had their sedation interrupted daily, but only after the administration of paralytic drugs had also been temporarily discontinued prior to sedative interruption. In both the intervention and control groups, all other clinical decisions and medication adjustments were left to the discretion of the intensive care unit team.

Follow-Up: Until hospital discharge or death.

Endpoints: Primary outcomes: duration of mechanical ventilation, length of ICU stay, length of hospital stay. Secondary outcomes: total dose of sedative (midazolam or propofol), morphine, and average infusion rates; percentage of days awake; use of neurologic tests; numbers of patients requiring paralytic drugs, reintubation, noninvasive ventilation, or tracheostomy; adverse events (e.g. self-extubation), transfer to a facility for long-term ventilation, transition of care to comfort, and in-hospital mortality.

RESULTS

- Patients who had daily sedation interruptions required fewer days of mechanical ventilation (4.9 vs. 7.3 days, $p = 0.004$) and had shorter stays in the ICU (6.4 vs. 9.9 days, $p = 0.02$) compared with the standard care group.
- The total dose of midazolam was lower in the daily awakening group than in the control group among the patients receiving midazolam, as was the total dose of morphine. In contrast, among the patients receiving propofol, there were no significant differences between the intervention and the control groups in the total dose of propofol or the total dose of morphine.
- Fewer diagnostic tests to assess changes in mental status (computer tomography, CT; magnetic resonance imagery, MRI; lumbar puncture) were performed in the daily awakening group than in the control group.
- There were no significant differences between the two groups in the number of adverse events or mortality rates.
- There were no significant differences between the two groups in the number of patients requiring reintubation, that underwent tracheostomy, or that were transferred to a long-term ventilation facility (Table 3.1).

Table 3.1. SUMMARY OF PRIMARY OUTCOMES

	Daily sedation interruption	Standard care	P Value
Duration of mechanical ventilation	4.9 days	7.3 days	0.004
Duration of ICU stay	6.4 days	9.9 days	0.02
Duration of hospitalization	13.3 days	16.9 days	0.19

Criticisms and Limitations:

- Despite the best efforts, it seems unlikely that the treating clinicians would be blinded to the study intervention, a fact acknowledged by the investigators. The lack of physician blinding could bias the results toward positive outcomes.
- The trial was limited to the medical intensive care unit so the results may not generalizable to other intensive care unit settings (e.g., surgical or neurosurgical patients).

- A major premise of the trial is that daily interruption of sedation is safe, but there are not enough patients included to be confident that the strategies have similar risk profiles. In particular, there does not appear to be any analysis of the psychological impacts of the study on the patients, their families, or on the nursing staff caring for them; however, a follow-up study reported a reduced incidence of post-traumatic stress disorder in the daily interruption group compared to control. The analyses in that study were done by psychologists blinded to patient randomization group.[2]
- Some critically ill patients have a hyperadrenergic stress response when sedation is reduced. The impact that a sudden interruption of sedation might have on myocardial oxygen balance in patients at risk for cardiac disease was not assessed; however, a follow-up study reported no difference in myocardial ischemia between the two groups.[3]
- This target sedation level in the control group (Ramsay Sedation Score of 3–4) may have been deeper than current ICU practice. Therefore the results may not be generalizable to ICUs that target lighter levels of sedation.

Other Relevant Studies and Information: A number of subsequent randomized trials and meta-analyses have reported benefit from daily interruption with regard to reducing duration of mechanical ventilation and length of stay. However, there is considerable heterogeneity among trials, which limits interpretation of the analysis. As examples:

- A Danish single-center trial demonstrated that a practice of no sedation compared to sedation with daily interruption resulted in significantly reduced time on a ventilator, days in the ICU, and days in the hospital.[4] Of note in the trial was the finding that agitated delirium was more frequent in the no-sedation group than in the daily interruption group.
- A Cochrane systematic review failed to find strong evidence that daily sedation interruption alters the duration of mechanical ventilation, mortality, length of ICU or hospital stay, or quality of life for critically ill adults receiving mechanical ventilation compared to sedation strategies without daily sedation interruption. However, the authors concluded that given the heterogeneity identified in the trials, the results should be considered "unstable rather than negative."[5]
- Adverse psychological effects related to daily sedation interruption have not been demonstrated. In fact, the inability to recall events in the ICU resulting from heavy sedation has been linked to the development of post-traumatic stress disorder.[2]

- The cardiovascular effects of daily sedation interruption were studied in prospective cohort study of patients with risk factors for coronary artery disease. although heart rate, blood pressure, respiratory rate, and catecholamines increased significantly during sedation interruption, myocardial ischemia was not more common.[3]
- The 2008 Awakening and Breathing Controlled Trial evaluated a "wake up and breathe" protocol that combined daily sedation holidays with spontaneous breathing trials (SBT).[6] This technique shortened the duration of mechanical ventilation, days in the ICU, and days in the hospital when compared to usual sedation techniques and daily SBTs. The concept has now been progressively expanded to the "ABCDE" approach—awake, breathing control, delirium assessment and early exercise model. This approach is recommended by the Society of Critical Care Medicine.[7]

Summary and Implications: This was the first trial to demonstrate that daily sedation interruption for mechanically ventilated medical ICU patients is safe and may reduce duration of mechanical ventilation and length of ICU stay. Subsequent studies suggest that protocol-driven sedation weaning may also be an effective strategy for weaning sedation safely and may similarly reduce duration of mechanical ventilation.

CLINICAL CASE: DAILY SEDATION INTERRUPTION IN THE INTENSIVE CARE UNIT

Case History:
A 68-year-old woman with chronic obstructive pulmonary disease and diabetes is admitted to the intensive care unit with septic shock and intubated for hypoxemic respiratory failure. After intubation she is agitated despite receiving appropriate amounts of opioids, so she is started on a sedative infusion of propofol infusion with a RASS goal of 0 (alert and calm) to –1 (drowsy). Based on the results of the trial by Kress et al., how should this patient be managed?

Suggested Answer:
Kress et al. showed that a daily interruption of sedative infusions decreases the duration of mechanical ventilation and ICU length of stay, as well as the need for neurodiagnostic testing for changes in mental status. The patient in this vignette is less sedated than patients in the conventional treatment arm of the study and in fact may be awake enough to follow commands, which

was the goal for sedation interruption in the study. Consequently the benefits of daily sedation interruption for this patient are unclear. For a patient that requires a deeper level of sedation (e.g., to achieve ventilator synchrony), daily interruption of sedation is likely to be beneficial.

References

1. Kress JP, Pohlman AS, O'Connor MF, Hall JB. Daily interruption of sedative infusions in critically ill patients undergoing mechanical ventilation. *N Engl J Med.*;342(20):1471–1477.
2. Kress JP, Gehlbach B, Lacy M, et al. The long-term psychological effects of daily sedative interruption on critically ill patients. *Am J Respir Crit Care Med.* 2003;168:1457.
3. Kress JP, Vinayak AG, Levitt J, et al. Daily sedative interruption in mechanically ventilated patients at risk for coronary artery disease. *Crit Care Med.* 2007;35:365.
4. Strøm T, Martinussen T, Toft P. A protocol of no sedation for critically ill patients receiving mechanical ventilation: a randomised trial. *Lancet.* 2010; 375(9713):475–480.
5. Burry L, Rose L, McCullagh IJ, Fergusson DA, Ferguson ND, Mehta S. Daily sedation interruption versus no daily sedation interruption for critically ill adult patients requiring invasive mechanical ventilation. *Cochrane Database Syst Rev.* 2014;(7):CD009176.
6. Girard TD, et al. Efficacy and safety of a paired sedation and ventilator weaning protocol for mechanically ventilated patients in intensive care (Awakening and Breathing Controlled trial): a randomised controlled trial. *Lancet.* 2008;371(9607):126–134.
7. Barr J, Fraser GL, Puntillo K, et al. Clinical practice guidelines for the management of pain, agitation, and delirium in adult patients in the intensive care unit. *Crit Care Med.* 2013;41(1):263–306.

4

A Comparison of Four Treatments
for Generalized Convulsive Status Epilepticus

JASON L. SANDERS AND JARONE LEE

"As initial intravenous treatment for overt generalized convulsive status epilepticus, lorazepam is more effective than phenytoin. Although lorazepam is no more efficacious than phenobarbital or diazepam and phenytoin, it is easier to use."

—TREIMAN DM, ET AL.

Research Question: Should patients with generalized convulsive status epilepticus be initially managed with intravenous diazepam followed by phenytoin, lorazepam, phenobarbital, or phenytoin?[1]

Funding: Department of Veterans Affairs Medical Research Services Cooperative Studies Program; Wyeth-Ayerst Laboratories

Year Study Began: 1990

Year Study Published: 1998

Study Location: 16 Veterans Affairs medical centers and 6 affiliated university hospitals in the United States

Who Was Studied: Two groups: (1) Patients with overt GCSE, defined as recurrent convulsions without complete recovery between seizures; (2) Patients

with subtle GCSE, defined as the stage of GCSE when the patient is in continuous coma but only subtle motor convulsions are seen.

Who Was Excluded: Patients who had received treatment and whose seizures
had stopped before enrollment; status epilepticus type other than generalized
convulsive; age less than 18 years; pregnancy; neurologic emergency requiring
immediate surgical intervention; presence of specific contraindications to therapy with hydantoin, benzodiazepine, or barbiturate drugs.

How Many Patients: 1705 patients were screened; 570 enrolled in intention-
to-treat analysis; of those, 518 with verified diagnosis of GCSE.

Study Overview: See Figure 4.1 for an overview of the study design.

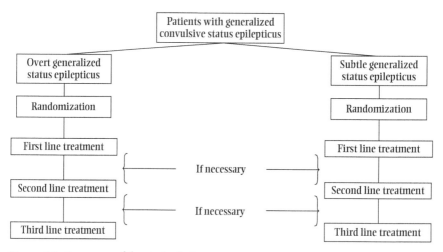

Figure 4.1 Summary of the study design.

Study Intervention: Randomized, double-blinded assignment of patients
to a first-line intervention of diazepam (0.15 mg/kg) followed by phenytoin
(18 mg/kg); lorazepam (0.1 mg/kg); phenobarbital (15 mg/kg); or phenytoin
(18 mg/kg). Phenytoin, phenobarbital, and diazepam were packaged in identical
vials at appropriate concentrations so each drug could be administered at a rate
of 1 mL/min to produce the maximal rate of drug infusion. Lorazepam was similarly packaged to produce the maximal infusion rate of 0.5 mL/min. If the seizure
did not cease after a first-line treatment box was given, providers progressed to
a second- and third-line treatment box, as needed, each containing active drug.
Treatment box regimens were randomized in a scheme to preserve balanced
groups according to intention-to-treat analysis.

Follow-Up: 12 hours after treatment

Endpoints: Primary outcome: If all clinical and electrical evidence of seizure activity stopped within 20 minutes after the start of the infusion and did not recur during the period from 20 to 60 minutes after the start of treatment. Secondary outcomes: outcome at 30 days; incidence of adverse reactions.

RESULTS

- Among patients with verified-diagnosis overt GCSE, lorazepam was most successful at achieving cessation of seizures (64.9%), followed by phenobarbital (58.2%), diazepam and phenytoin (55.8%), and phenytoin (43.6%; $p = 0.02$ across all groups).
- Among patients with verified-diagnosis subtle GCSE, no significant difference in treatment success was observed: phenobarbital 24.2%, lorazepam 17.9%, diazepam and phenytoin 8.3%, phenytoin 7.7% ($p = 0.18$ across all groups). Notably, none of the patients with subtle GCSE completely regained consciousness during the 12-hour study period.
- There were no differences among the treatments in the frequency of recurrence of overt or subtle status epilepticus during the 12-hour study period, suggesting that any of the four treatments, if successful, can protect equally well against recurrence. There were no significant differences across treatment groups in outcome at 30 days, or in incidence of adverse reactions.

Criticisms and Limitations:

- Diagnostic criteria for status epilepticus have changed. The duration of seizure required for status epilepticus used in the study was 10 minutes, which differs from the definition of 5 minutes used in recent years. In addition, the definition of subtle convulsive status epilepticus probably included a population of what is now called non-convulsive status epilepticus, as the criteria in the study was "with or without subtle convulsive movements.
- The population was predominantly male, thus limiting the study's generalizability to other subgroups.
- Results may not apply to seizures of types other than GCSE, or seizures in children, pregnant patients, or patients requiring emergent surgical interventions (e.g., seizures with traumatic brain injury).

- Treatment superiority may be confounded by allowable maximum infusion rates. Because lorazepam infuses faster than phenytoin, lorazepam achieves therapeutic levels more quickly. Nonetheless, this represents real-world conditions, which may make lorazepam more efficacious for an emergent condition that requires rapid entry of drug into the brain.
- Treatment superiority may be confounded by the length of time between start of seizure and administration of drug. Seizures that begin in the field may be treated immediately by adjacent caregivers (e.g., parents administering rectal midazolam to a seizing child), quickly by paramedics (e.g., intramuscular midazolam or intravenous lorazepam), or with greater delay in an emergency department. Seizures that begin in a hospitalized patient may be treated rapidly with several drugs via several routes of administration.
- Detection of seizure cessation may require continuous electrical monitoring of brain activity. Equipment or rapid interpretation of its recordings may not be readily available to providers. This complicates real-world practice when decisions must be made about whether to continue with a certain drug, add another anti-epileptic drug, or switch drug classes.
- Newer antiepileptic drugs have become widespread. These include fosphenytoin, which has fewer side effects and can be infused more rapidly than phenytoin; levetiracetam, which has few drug-drug interactions and side effects and does not require weight-based dosing or monitoring of levels; propofol, which has strong anti-epileptic effects, can facilitate induction for intubation, and can be used for long-term sedation but additionally requires intubation and can cause significant hypotension; as well as valproic acid and lacosamide.

Other Relevant Studies and Information:

- Out-of-hospital treatment by paramedics of status epilepticus in adults using benzodiazepines versus placebo was effective and safe and favored lorazepam compared to diazepam.[2]
- Intravenous access may be difficult to obtain in the field, particularly in a seizing patient. In a double-blind, randomized, non-inferiority trial of intramuscular midazolam versus intravenous lorazepam administered in the field by paramedics to seizing children and adults, midazolam was at least as effective and safe as lorazepam, and had a median time to treatment of 1.2 minutes versus 4.8 minutes.[3]
- One third of patients with status epilepticus continue to have seizures despite treatment with benzodiazepines. There are no randomized

trials to guide treatment in benzodiazepine-refractory status epilepticus (established status epilepticus). The Established Status Epilepticus Trial will compare fosphenytoin, levetiracetam, and valproic acid in a multicenter, randomized, double-blind, Bayesian adaptive, phase III comparative effectiveness trial, including patients older than 2 years.[4]

• Guidelines from the American Epilepsy Society recommend a benzodiazepine (specifically IM midazolam, IV lorazepam, or IV diazepam) as the initial therapy of choice for status epilepticus, given their demonstrated efficacy, safety, and tolerability. Although IV phenobarbital is established as efficacious and well tolerated as initial therapy, its slower rate of administration, compared with the three recommended benzodiazepines above, positions it as an alternative initial therapy.[5]

Summary and Implications: Among patients presenting with undifferentiated GCSE, it is reasonable to administer intravenous lorazepam at a dose of 0.1 mg/kg as the first line agent for cessation of seizures, compared to diazepam and phenytoin, phenobarbital, or phenytoin. Treatment superiority at 30 days is unclear. Adverse side effects are similar across treatments. These results do not necessarily apply to seizures of types other than GCSE, or seizures in children, pregnant patients, or patients requiring emergent surgical intervention.

CLINICAL CASE: GENERALIZED CONVULSIVE STATUS EPILEPTICUS

Case History:
A 50-year-old male with hypertension, hyperlipidemia, and a substantial smoking history has been a patient on the general medical service for two days for treatment of pneumonia. He has a witnessed generalized convulsive seizure with an intervening post-ictal state from which he never completely recovers and subsequently begins seizing again. Based on the results of the Veterans Affairs Status Epilepticus Cooperative Study Group, how should this patient be treated?

Suggested Answer:
This patient's seizure initially stopped, but he never completely recovered, progressing from an isolated seizure to GCSE. The preferred first line treatment is lorazepam 0.1 mg/kg at an infusion rate of 0.5 mg/min. If he fails to respond to lorazepam, phenobarbital may be the next most appropriate therapy.

References

1. Treiman DM, Meyers PD, Walton NY, et al. A comparison of four treatments for generalized convulsive status epilepticus. Veterans Affairs Status Epilepticus Cooperative
   Study Group. *N Engl J Med.* 1998;339(12):792–798.
2. Alldredge BK, Gelb AM, Isaacs SM, et al. A comparison of lorazepam, diazepam,
   and placebo for the treatment of out-of-hospital status epilepticus. *N Engl J Med.*
   2001;345(9):631–637.
3. Silbergleit R, Durkalski V, Lowenstein D, et al. Intramuscular versus intravenous therapy for prehospital status epilepticus. *N Engl J Med.* 2012;366(7):591–600.
4. Bleck T, Cock H, Chamberlain J, et al. The established status epilepticus trial 2013.
   Epilepsia. 2013;54 Suppl 6:89–92.
5. Glauser T, Shinnar S, Gloss D, et al. Evidence-based guideline: treatment of convulsive status epilepticus in children and adults: report of the Guideline Committee of
   the American Epilepsy Society. *Epilepsy Curr.* 2016;16(1):48–61.

5

Efficacy and Safety of a Paired Sedation and Ventilator Weaning Protocol for Mechanically Ventilated Patients in Intensive Care

A Randomized Controlled Trial (The ABC Trial)

JEFFERY KATZ AND STEVE GREENBERG

"A so called wake up and breathe protocol that pairs daily spontaneous awakening trials with daily spontaneous breathing trials for the management of mechanically ventilated patients in intensive care results in better outcomes than current standard approaches . . . "

—GIRARD ET AL.

Research Question: For patients requiring mechanical ventilation is there a benefit of pairing daily sedation awakening trials with spontaneous breathing trials?[1]

Funding: Saint Thomas Foundation; National Institutes of Health; Veterans Affairs Tennessee Valley Geriatric Research, Education, and Clinical Center; the Hartford Geriatrics Health Outcomes Research Scholars Award Program; and the Vanderbilt Physician Scientist Development Program.

Year Study Began: 2003

Year Study Published: 2008

Study Location: Four large medical centers: Saint Thomas Hospital (Nashville, TN), University of Chicago Hospitals (Chicago, IL), Hospital of the University of Pennsylvania (Philadelphia, PA), and Penn Presbyterian Medical Center (Philadelphia, PA).

Who Was Studied: Patients older than 18 years requiring mechanical ventilation in the intensive care unit (ICU) for at least 12 hours who were eligible for weaning.

Who Was Excluded: Patients admitted for cardiac arrest, greater than 2 weeks of mechanical ventilation, neurologic dysfunction, moribund state, or enrollment in another trial. Surgical patients were also excluded from this trial.

How Many Patients: 336

Study Overview: See Figure 5.1 for an overview of the study's design.

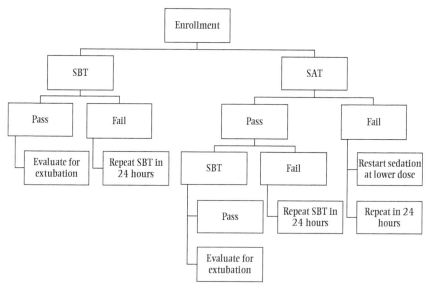

Figure 5.1 ABC Trial Study Design. Adapted from Girard, et al.[1]

Study Intervention: Patients enrolled in the control group ("the spontaneous breathing arm") underwent a protocolized spontaneous breathing trial (SBT) each morning. The SBT included standard ventilator weaning modes including T-piece, continuous positive airway pressure (CPAP) 5 cm H_2O, or pressure support ventilation with inspiratory pressure less than 7 cm H_2O). If a patient failed the SBT, the previous ventilator settings were reinitiated. If a patient passed the SBT, the ICU team was notified.

Patients enrolled in the intervention group (the "wake up and breathe" arm) had a daily spontaneous awakening trial (SAT). Patients who failed the SAT had their sedation resumed at half the previous dose. If the patient passed the SAT, they had an SBT using the same protocol as patients in the control arm.

Follow-Up: 1 year

Endpoints:

- *Primary Outcome*: Ventilator-free days
- *Secondary Outcomes:* Time to discharge from ICU, time to discharge from hospital, 28 day mortality, 1 year mortality, duration of coma, duration of delirium, Richmond Agitation-Sedation Scale (RASS) Score at first successful spontaneous breathing trial (SBT), self extubation, self-extubation requiring re-intubation, re-intubation, tracheostomy.

RESULTS

- The two groups did not differ in their baseline characteristics, including age, sex, diagnosis on admission to the ICU, APACHE II, or SOFA scores. The intervention group did receive a higher dose of propofol prior to enrollment in the study, but there were no differences in the doses of benzodiazepines or opiates. Patients in the intervention ("wake up and breathe") group spent on average 3.1 more days liberated from the ventilator compared with the control group.
- Patients in the "wake up and breathe" group were discharged from the ICU a median of 3.8 days earlier than the control group. Similarly, the patients in the intervention group were discharged from the hospital a median of 4 days earlier than the control group.
- There was no statistical difference in 28-day survival; however, at one year the patients in the intervention group were 32% more likely to be alive than the control group.
- More patients in the "wake up and breathe" group self-extubated than in the control group, but the number of patients who required reintubation was similar in both groups.
- The duration of coma was shorter in the "wake up and breathe" group when compared to the control group, but no difference was found in the incidence of delirium (Table 5.1).

Table 5.1. SUMMARY OF KEY FINDINGS

	"Wake Up and Breathe" Group	Control Group	*P* Value
Ventilator-free days	14.7 (0.9)	11.6 (0.9)	0.02
ICU length of stay (days)	9.1 (5.1 to 17.8)	12.9 (6.0 to 24.2)	0.01
One year mortality	44%	58%	0.01

Criticisms and Limitations:

- The ABC Trial did not include surgical patients, and the generalizability of the study's findings to this population is unknown. The need for continuous analgesia in surgical patients may alter the results of a paired daily awakening and spontaneous breathing trial.
- The study was performed at large academic centers with adequate staffing of nurses and respiratory therapists. This study's finding may not be applicable to centers that do not have these staffing characteristics.
- Although randomized, the trial was not blinded, which may have introduced bias.
- The trial did not specifically and prospectively investigate the impact of each approach on cognition, psychological, or functional outcomes associated with coupling SAT with SBT.

Other Relevant Studies and Information:

1. Daily assessment of respiratory function and spontaneous breathing trials in mechanically ventilated patients may facilitate faster liberation from mechanical ventilation.[2]
2. There is evidence of reduced duration of mechanical ventilation, weaning duration, and ICU length of stay with use of standardized weaning protocols.[3] However, for mechanically ventilated adults managed with protocolized sedation, the addition of daily sedation interruption does not appear to reduce the duration of mechanical ventilation or ICU stay.[4]
3. An a priori, planned substudy conducted at one hospital participating in the ABC trial reported similar cognitive, psychological, and functional outcomes among patients tested 3 and 12 months post-ICU in both the intervention and control groups.[5]
4. Barriers to implementation of paired sedation and ventilator weaning protocols may exist in actual clinical practice that limit their efficacy.[6]
5. Recently the addition of delirium monitoring and management, "D," and early mobility and exercise, "E," have been added to the ABC

protocol, forming the ABCDE bundle as a strategy for improving ICU outcomes. The ABCDE has been proposed a (Awakening and Breathing Coordination of daily sedation and ventilator removal trials; Choice of sedative or analgesic exposure; Delirium monitoring and management; and Early mobility and Exercise). While the effect of reliable ABCDE bundle adoption on the incidence and outcomes of PICS has yet to be fully studied, intuitively it is an extremely promising approach.[7]

Summary and Implications: In medical ICU patients, protocolization of daily sedation awakening trials with spontaneous breathing trials may significantly improve the outcomes of patients requiring mechanical ventilation including hospital and ICU length of stay and mortality.

CLINICAL CASE: USING THE ABC TRIAL

Case History:
A 75-year-old male with history significant for alcohol abuse has been admitted to the ICU with respiratory failure from pneumonia. He has been intubated and mechanically ventilated for the last 72 hours. His last drink was reportedly on the day of admission. His vital signs are BP 175/94, HR 110, O2 saturation 99% on 40% FiO2. Despite sedation with a propofol infusion he is diaphoretic and intermittently agitated. A medical student asks on rounds whether this patient is acceptable to proceed for a SAT and then a SBT. What would you tell him?

Suggested Answer:
This patient is probably not ready for a SAT. He has a history of alcohol abuse and signs/symptoms consistent with acute alcohol withdrawal. The ABC trial excluded patients with alcohol withdrawal given safety concern regarding abrupt cessation of benzodiazepines. Patients that have completed their alcohol withdrawal phase may be assessed on an individualized basis for SAT and SBT.

References

1. Girard TD, et al. Efficacy and safety of a paired sedation and ventilator weaning protocol for mechanically ventilated patients in intensive care (Awakening and Breathing Controlled trial): a randomised controlled trial. *Lancet.* 2008;371:126–134.
2. Ely EW, et al. Effect on the duration of mechanical ventilation of identifying patients capable of breathing spontaneously. *New Engl J Med.* 1996;335:1864–1869.

3. Blackwood B, Burns KE, Cardwell CR, O'Halloran P. Protocolized versus non-protocolized weaning for reducing the duration of mechanical ventilation in critically ill adult patients. *Cochrane Database Syst Rev.* 2014;11:CD006904.
4. Mehta S, Burry L, Cook D, et al.; SLEAP Investigators; Canadian Critical Care Trials Group. Daily sedation interruption in mechanically ventilated critically ill patients cared for with a sedation protocol: a randomized controlled trial. J Am Med Assoc. 2012;308(19):1985–1992.
5. Jackson JC, Girard T, Gordon SM, Thompson JL, et al. Long-term Cognitive and Psychological Outcomes in the Awakening and Breathing Controlled Trial. *Am J Respir Crit Care Med.* 2010;182: 183–191.
6. Kher S, Roberts RJ, Garpestad E, Kunkel C, Howard W, Didominico D, Fergusson A, Devlin JW. Development, implementation, and evaluation of an institutional daily awakening and spontaneous breathing trial protocol: a quality improvement project. *J Intensive Care Med.* 2013;28(3):189–197.
7. Pandharipande P, Banerjee A, McGrane S, Ely EW. Liberation and animation for ventilated ICU patients: the ABCDE bundle for the back-end of critical care. *Crit Care.* 2010;14(3):157.

6

A Protocol of No Sedation for Critically Ill Patients Receiving Mechanical Ventilation

A Randomized Trial

ULRICH SCHMIDT AND ZEB MCMILLAN

"No sedation of critically ill patients receiving mechanical ventilation is associated with an increase in days without ventilation."
—STROM T ET AL.

Research Question: Can duration of mechanical ventilation be reduced with a protocol of no sedation versus daily interruption of sedation?[1]

Year Study Published: 2010

Study Location: Odense University Hospital, Denmark

Who Was Studied: Critically ill adult patients (medical and surgical) undergoing mechanical ventilation and expected to need mechanical ventilation for more than 24 hours. Patients transferred intubated from other ICUs were also included.

Who Was Excluded: Patients with age < 18, increased ICP, needing sedation (e.g., for status epilepticus or hypothermia after cardiac arrest), pregnant, meeting criteria for weaning from ventilation ($FiO_2 \leq 40\%$ and positive end-expiratory pressure of 5 cm H_2O), or who had no cerebral contact (ex coma hepatica).

How Many Patients: 140 adult patients; 27 patients were excluded from analysis because mechanical ventilation was stopped within 48 hours.

Study Overview: See Figure 6.1 for an overview of the study design.

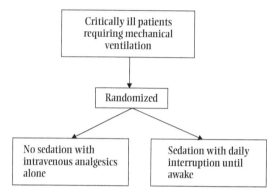

Figure 6.1 Summary of the study design.

Intervention: Within 24 hours after intubation, patients were randomly assigned to receive sedation with daily interruption until awake (control group), or no sedation with bolus intravenous analgesics alone (intervention group). Both groups received IV morphine in bolus doses (2.5 or 5 mg) as needed. For management of delirium, IV haloperidol was administered. If possible, patients in both groups were mobilized during daily interruption to a chair despite mechanical ventilation. The standard ventilation mode was pressure support unless severe prolonged hypoventilation was present. All patients were weaned from the ventilator based on a local weaning protocol.

- In the intervention group, if patients were uncomfortable a doctor assessed them for possible causes of discomfort. If needed, a person was assigned to verbally comfort and reassure the patient. If they still seemed uncomfortable, they were sedated with propofol for 6 hours, and then sedation was held and attempted to continue again without sedation. After 3 failed attempts at no sedation, the patient was kept sedated with daily interruptions as in the control group but remained in the intervention group for final analysis by intent to treat.
- The control group was sedated with a propofol infusion to achieve a Ramsay score of 3–4. Each day, sedation was interrupted until patients were awake and could follow simple commands. Sedation was then restarted at half the previous dose and titrated to a Ramsay score of 3–4. After 48 hours, the sedative was changed to an infusion of midazolam titrated to a Ramsay score of 3–4 and continued with daily interruptions until extubated. Sedation was stopped in the control group when the

ventilator settings reached FiO$_2$ 40% and PEEP of 5 cm H$_2$O, and they were treated as if they were in the intervention group in terms of sedation management, unless the FiO$_2$ increased above 50% or PEEP above 8 cm H$_2$O.

Follow-Up: 28 days from intubation.

Endpoints:

- Primary outcome: Number of ventilator-free days in a 28-day period.
- Secondary outcomes: Frequency of the need for CT or MRI brain scans, accidental removal of the endotracheal tube, and ventilator-associated pneumonia.
- Patients who had their endotracheal tube removed or died during the first 48 hours were not included in the analysis.

RESULTS

- The no-sedation group had more ventilator-free days compared to the group with continuous sedation (13.8 days vs. 9.6 days, $p = 0.0191$).
- Length of stay in the intensive care unit was significantly shorter in the no-sedation group than in the sedation group (13.1 vs. 22.8 days, $p = 0.0316$)
- Length of hospital stay was significantly shorter in the no-sedation group than in the sedation group.
- Mortality in the intensive care unit and in hospital overall was higher in the sedation group than in the no sedation group, but none of the differences reached statistical significance.
- There was no difference in the need for CT/MRI brain scans, ventilator-associated pneumonia, or reintubation within 24 hours.
- There was more agitated delirium in the no-sedation group than in the control group (20% vs. 7%; $p = 0.0400$). Haloperidol was administered more frequently in the intervention group (Table 6.1).

Table 6.1. SUMMARY OF THE STUDY'S KEY FINDINGS

	No Sedation	Sedation	*P* Value
Ventilator-free days Mean (SD)	13.8 (11.0)	9.6 (10.0)	0.0191
ICU length of stay (LOS) (median days)	13.1	22.8	0.0316
Hospital LOS (median days)	34	58	0.0039
In-hospital mortality	36%	47%	0.27

Criticisms and Limitations:

- The intervention of "no sedation" was the institution's standard practice, and together with the lack of blinding, may have resulted in bias in favor of the no-sedation group. In addition, external validity may be limited, as there may be a learning curve associated with using "no sedation."
- The study used a 1:1 nurse to patient ratio and patient comforters. The requirement for more staff presence is likely to be unavailable in most ICUs, which may limit generalizability.
- If patients still needed mechanical ventilation after 48 h, propofol was switched to midazolam for sedation, which has a longer clearance time and has been associated with increased duration of mechanical ventilation and longer ICU length of stay.[2]
- The intervention group had more agitated delirium. However, the detection of delirium was not a primary or secondary endpoint, and the presence of hypoactive delirium was not evaluated, which may have differed between groups.
- Post-traumatic stress disorder (PTSD) is commonly reported in survivors of critical illness and is an important outcome in studies that attempt to reduce sedation. However the prevalence of PTSD was not evaluated in this study.
- 18% of patients in the no-sedation group required continuous sedation. This highlights the difficulty with applying this no-sedation strategy despite expertise and staffing.
- A slightly increased severity of illness and SOFA score in the control group (SAPS II 46 vs. 50, and SOFA 7.5 vs. 9). This may have biased results toward the experimental group.

Other Relevant Studies and Information:

- In 2000, a single-center study by Kress et al. randomized 128 intubated ICU patients to either daily interruptions of sedation (commonly known as "sedation holidays") or interruptions when it was thought to be appropriate by the intensivist. Daily sedation holidays were associated with a decreased duration of mechanical ventilation by 2.8 days and time in the ICU by 3.5 days.[3]
- Continuous sedative infusions have been associated with longer duration of mechanical ventilation, longer intensive care unit (ICU) length of stay, ventilator-associated complications, delirium and posttraumatic stress disorder.[5]
- Subsequent studies have extended on the findings of the Kress et al trial. For example, the 2008 Awakening and Breathing Controlled

(ABC) Trial evaluated a "wake up and breathe" protocol that followed daily sedation holidays with spontaneous breathing trials (SBT). This technique reduced time on a ventilator, days in the ICU, and days in the hospital when compared to usual sedation techniques and daily SBTs.[5]

Randomized trials have not consistently replicated the impressive findings of Kress et al. A 2011 meta-analysis of 5 trials of sedation interruptions did not show that sedation holidays reduced ventilator-days among 699 patients, although it did seem safe (no excess self-extubations) and led to fewer tracheostomies.[6]

- A follow-up study suggests that a protocol of no sedation in critically ill patients undergoing mechanical ventilation does not increase the risk of long-term psychological sequelae compared with standard sedation treatment.[7]
- The Society of Critical Care Medicine's 2013 Pain, Agitation, and Delirium (PAD) Guidelines recommend daily sedation interruption or light target level of sedation for adult ICU patients on mechanical ventilation. In addition, the PAD guidelines suggest sedation using non-benzodiazepine sedatives (propofol or dexmedetomidine) for adult ICU patients on mechanical ventilation.[8]

Summary and Implications: In critically ill patients receiving mechanical ventilation, a protocol of no sedation appears to increase the number of ventilator-free days compared with daily interruption of sedation. A strategy of "no sedation" may be feasible in ICUs, but may require additional staffing to ensure patient safety. Larger, multicenter trials are needed to confirm the findings of this study and to evaluate the impact of no sedation on long term patient centered outcomes.

CLINICAL CASE: A PROTOCOL OF NO SEDATION FOR CRITICALLY ILL PATIENTS RECEIVING MECHANICAL VENTILATION: A RANDOMIZED TRIAL

Case History:

A 55-year-old man with COPD and a 15 pack/year smoking history is admitted to the ICU with respiratory failure and sepsis due to community acquired pneumonia. His most recent ABG shows a pH of 7.30, pCO_2 of 33, PaO_2 of 190 mm Hg, and a bicarbonate of 19 mEq/L on volume control ventilation with a tidal volume of 450 mL, PEEP of 5, and an FiO_2 of 50%. His vital signs on ICU admission are BP 130/70, HR 95, and Temp 36.1. The nurse asks you if you would like the patient to have a midazolam drip for sedation overnight with morphine for pain. Based on the results of the study, is this an appropriate sedation regimen?

Suggested Answer:

Understanding that not all patients receiving mechanical ventilation require sedation is an important first step to deciding what regimen is best for this patient. Based on the results of the study, a strategy of less sedation appears to be beneficial in terms of reducing ventilator days and does not appear to cause harm when adequate levels of staffing are available. If the patient appears comfortable, no additional sedatives are necessary. If the patient appears uncomfortable, the patient should be evaluated to discover the source of discomfort. Previous studies have also shown that infusions of benzodiazepine are associated with increases in the duration of mechanical ventilation and ICU length of stay and therefore should be avoided. If needed, short-acting sedatives such as propofol or dexmedetomidine are probably better than benzodiazepines. It is important to treat pain prior to increasing levels of sedation and to regularly reassess for the need for sedation.

References

1. Strom T, Martinussen T, Toft P: A protocol of no sedation for critically ill patients receiving mechanical ventilation: a randomized trial. *Lancet.* 2010;375:475–480.
2. Fraser GL, Devlin JW, Worby CP, Alhazzani W, Barr J, Dasta JF, Kress JP, Davidson JE, Spencer FA. Benzodiazepine versus nonbenzodiazepine-based sedation for mechanically ventilated, critically ill adults: a systematic review and meta-analysis of randomized trials. *Crit Care Med.* 2013;41(9 Suppl 1):S30–38.
3. Kress JP, Pohlman AS, O'Connor MF, Hall JB: Daily interruption of sedative infusions in critically ill patients undergoing mechanical ventilation. *N Engl J Med.* 2000;342:1471–1477.
4. Kollef MH, Levy NT, Ahrens TS, Schaiff R, Prentice D, Sherman G: The use of continuous i.v. sedation is associated with prolongation of mechanical ventilation. *Chest.* 1998;114:541–548.
5. Girard TD, Kress JP, Fuchs BD, et al Efficacy and safety of a paired sedation and ventilator weaning protocol for mechanically ventilated patients in intensive care (Awakening and Breathing Controlled trial): a randomised controlled trial. Lancet. 2008;371(9607):126–134.
6. Augustes R, Ho KM. Meta-analysis of randomised controlled trials on daily sedation interruption for critically ill adult patients. *Anaesth Intensive Care.* 2011;39(3):401–4099.
7. Strøm T, Stylsvig M, Toft P. Psychological long-term effects of a no-sedation protocol in critically ill patients. *Crit Care.* 2011;15(Suppl 1): P359.
8. Barr J, Fraser GL, Puntillo K, et al. Clinical practice guidelines for the management of pain, agitation, and delirium in adult patients in the intensive care unit. *Crit Care Med.* 2013;41(1):263–306.

7

Intracranial Pressure Monitoring in Severe Traumatic Brain Injury

THOMAS PEPONIS AND DAVID R. KING

"Our results do not support the hypothesized superiority of management guided by intracranial-pressure monitoring over management guided by neurologic examination and serial CT imaging in patients with severe traumatic brain injury."

—CHESNUT ET AL.

Research Question: Does management based on intracranial-pressure (ICP) monitoring lead to diminished mortality and improved neuropsychological and functional recovery at six months following a severe traumatic brain injury (TBI)?[1]

Funding: The National Institutes of Health, the Fogarty International Center, the National Institute of Neurologic Disorders and Stroke, and Integra Life Sciences.

Year Study Began: 2008

Year Study Published: 2012

Study Location: 4 hospitals in Bolivia and 2 hospitals in Ecuador

Who Was Studied: Patients older than 13 years of age presenting with TBI and a Glasgow Coma Scale (GCS) ≤ 8 (with a GCS motor score of 1 to 5 if the patient was intubated). Patients who had a greater GCS on admission were also eligible, if the GSC deteriorated to between 3 and 8, within 48 hours post-injury.

Who Was Excluded: Patients with a GCS of 3 and bilateral fixed and dilated pupils, plus those whose injury was deemed unsurvivable.

How Many Patients: 324

Study Overview: Patients admitted with severe TBI were randomly assigned to two groups (Figure 7.1).

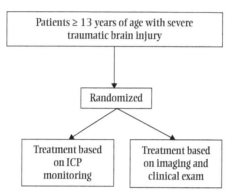

Figure 7.1 Summary of the study design.

Study Intervention: All patients were aggressively resuscitated and managed in ICU under close supervision by intensivists with a strong interest in TBI. Patients admitted with severe TBI were randomly assigned to two groups. The "pressure-monitoring" group was managed with ICP monitoring, using an intraparenchymal monitor. The goal was to keep the ICP ≤ 20 mm Hg. Management of patients in the "clinical examination-imaging" group was based solely on serial clinical examination and imaging tests. Signs of intracranial hypertension were treated using sedation, analgesia, and hyperosmolar agents. Hyperventilation (goal PCO_2 between 30 and 35 mm Hg) and ventricular drainage were used at the discretion of the treating clinicians. Finally, decompressive craniectomy and high-dose barbiturates were reserved for cases with evidence of persistent edema.

Follow-Up: The patients were assessed by blinded examiners at 3 and 6 months following the head injury.

Endpoints: Primary outcome was a composite of survival time, duration and level of impaired consciousness, functional status and orientation 3 months after the injury, plus functional and neuropsychological status at 6 months after the injury. Secondary outcomes were ICU length of stay and systemic complications.

RESULTS

- There was no significant difference between the pressure-monitoring group versus the imaging–clinical examination groups with respect to the primary outcome, a composite measure based on survival, duration and level of impaired consciousness, functional status and orientation 3 months after injury, and functional and neuropsychological status 6 months after injury.
- There was no significant difference in 6-month mortality, length of ICU stay, or duration of mechanical ventilation in the pressure-monitoring group versus the imaging–clinical examination groups.
- The number of patients undergoing neurosurgical procedures, such as craniectomies, did not differ between the groups.
- The number of days of brain-specific treatments (e.g., administration of hyperosmolar fluids and the use of hyperventilation) administered in the ICU was higher in the imaging–clinical examination group than in the pressure-monitoring group (Table 7.1).

Table 7.1. SUMMARY OF THE STUDY'S KEY FINDINGS

Outcome	ICP-Monitoring Group	Imaging/Clinical Examination Group	*P* value
Primary outcome (median composite score)	56	53	0.49
6-month mortality rate	39%	41%	0.60
14-day mortality rate	21%	30%	0.18
ICU length of stay (days)	12	9	0.25
Hospital length of stay (days)	**24**	**20**	**0.04**
Non-neurologic complications	134 (85%)	147 (88%)	0.52
Decubitus ulcers	**19 (12%)**	**8 (5%)**	**0.03**

Criticisms and Limitations:

- The study did not test the utility of ICP monitoring directly. It investigated the use of ICP data to drive an accepted management protocol as applied to all severe TBI patients. The results apply more to the method in which ICP is currently interpreted and treated than to the role of ICP monitoring itself in TBI care.
- The study was relatively small and may have been underpowered for detecting modest differences between the groups. Thus it is possible small benefits from ICP monitoring were not identified in this study.

- The study was conducted in two developing countries; hence, the generalization of results to other populations may be limited. Pre-hospital management of trauma patients may be suboptimal in these countries, and as a result severely injured patients may have passed away en route to the hospital. Subsequently, they may have been underrepresented.
- Notably, 35% of the mortality is attributed to deaths occurring after the first 2 weeks. The fact that rehabilitation services and continuing medical care after discharge in these countries are limited may be responsible for this relatively large percentage. Survival rates at 6 months may have been confounded by this phenomenon.
- The median age of patients in the study is 29 years. This does not reflect the reality in high-income countries, where the majority of patients admitted with severe TBIs are significantly older.

Other Relevant Studies and Information:

- Other studies have also failed to show a survival benefit in patients with severe TBI managed with ICP-monitoring.[2] In fact, a retrospective study[3] showed a decrease in survival among patients managed with ICP-monitoring.
- Two recently published, nonrandomized prospective studies suggest that ICP-monitoring in patients with severe TBI results in a survival benefit.[5,6]
- A large meta-analysis,[7] comprising 14 studies (24,792 patients), showed no significant difference in survival rates between ICP and non-ICP monitoring in patients with TBI. However, both ICU and hospital length of stay were significantly longer in the ICP-monitoring group. Importantly, however, among 7 studies published after 2012 (12,944 patients), ICP-monitoring led to decreased mortality rates.
- Guidelines for the Brain Trauma Foundation recommend using information from ICP monitoring for management of patients with severe TBI.[8]

Summary and Implications: This trial failed to demonstrate a significant benefit from ICP-based treatment versus treatment guided by serial clinical examinations and imaging among patients with severe TBI. The role of ICP monitoring among such patients remains a matter of debate.

CLINICAL CASE: ICP-MONITORING IN SEVERE TRAUMATIC BRAIN INJURY

Case History:

A 42-year-old male is transferred to your Level I Trauma Center after being involved in a motor vehicle collision. Vital signs are within normal limits and stable both in the field and the ED bay. On presentation, the patient's GCS is 5 and he is intubated. His brain CT scan demonstrates a frontal lobe intraparenchymal hemorrhage and a 12 mm subdural hematoma. There is 6 mm midline shift and compressed mesencephalic cisterns. Following urgent surgical evacuation his GCS remains 5. How should you manage this patient?

Suggested Answer:

Despite the results of this study, the accumulated evidence together with current guidelines suggest that this patient should be managed with ICP monitoring. The very low GCS and the severe head injury burden are compelling reasons to consider this management option. Intraoperatively, an intraventricular monitor can be easily placed. The ethical obstacles of not placing a monitor on such a patient would be difficult to overcome, especially in a high-income country. Additionally, he should have a neck CTA to exclude blunt cerebrovascular injury, as the cause of the persistently low GCS.

References

1. Chesnut RM, Temkin N, Carney N, et al. A trial of intracranial-pressure monitoring in traumatic brain injury. *N Engl J Med.* 2012;367(26):2471–2481.
2. Cremer OL, van Dijk GW, van Wensen E, et al. Effect of intracranial pressure monitoring and targeted intensive care on functional outcome after severe head injury. *Crit Care Med.* 2005;33(10):2207–2213.
3. Shafi S, Diaz-Arrastia R, Madden C, Gentilello L. Intracranial pressure monitoring in brain-injured patients is associated with worsening of survival. *J Trauma.* 2008;64(2):335–340.
4. The Brain Trauma Foundation. The American Association of Neurological Surgeons. The Joint Section on Neurotrauma and Critical Care. Indications for intracranial pressure monitoring. *J Neurotrauma.* 2000;17(6–7):479–91.
5. Dawes AJ, Sacks GD, Cryer HG, et al. Intracranial pressure monitoring and inpatient mortality in severe traumatic brain injury: a propensity score-matched analysis. *J Trauma Acute Care Surg.* 2015;78(3):492–501.

6. Farahvar A, Gerber LM, Chiu YL, Carney N, Härtl R, Ghajar J. Increased mortality in patients with severe traumatic brain injury treated without intracranial pressure monitoring. *J Neurosurg.* 2012;117(4):729–734.

7. Yuan Q, Wu X, Sun Y, et al. Impact of intracranial pressure monitoring on mortality in patients with traumatic brain injury: a systematic review and meta-analysis. *J Neurosurg.* 2015;122(3):574–587.

8. Carney N, Totten AM, O'Reilly C, et al. Guidelines for the Management of Severe Traumatic Brain Injury, Fourth Edition. *Neurosurgery.* 2017;80(1):6–15.

Cardiovascular, Resuscitation, Shock

8

Early Goal-Directed Therapy in the Treatment of Severe Sepsis and Septic Shock

The EGDT Trial

NAMITA JAYAPRAKASH AND JOSEPH HYDER

"Early goal-directed therapy provides significant benefits with respect to outcome in patients with severe sepsis and septic shock."

—RIVERS ET AL., 2001

Research Question: Among patients with severe sepsis or septic shock, does early goal-directed therapy (EGDT) reduce the incidence of multi-organ dysfunction, mortality, and the use of health care resources?[1]

Sponsor: Henry Ford Health Systems Fund for Research. There was no extramural funding or industrial support. All catheters were bought from Edwards Lifesciences and lactate levels performed by Nova Biomedical.

Year Study Began: 1997

Year Study Published: 2001

Study Overview: See Figure 8.1 for an overview of the study design.

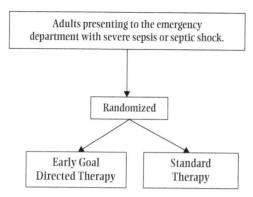

Figure 8.1 Summary of the study design.

Study Location: Emergency Department of a single 850-bed academic tertiary care hospital.

Who Was Studied: Adults presenting to the emergency department who fulfilled 2 of 4 criteria of the systemic inflammatory response syndrome (SIRS) criteria. They were also required to have a systolic blood pressure no greater than 90 mm Hg (after crystalloid fluid challenge) or a blood lactate concentration of ≥ 4 mmoL/L.

Who Was Excluded: Patients were excluded if there was an acute cerebral vascular event, acute coronary syndrome, acute pulmonary edema, status asthmaticus, cardiac dysrhythmias (as a primary diagnosis), contraindication to central venous catheterization, active gastrointestinal hemorrhage, seizure, drug overdose, burn injury, trauma, a requirement for immediate surgery, uncured cancer (during chemotherapy), immunosuppression (because of organ transplantation or systemic disease), do-not-resuscitate status, or advanced directives restricting implementation of the protocol.

How Many Patients: 263

Study Intervention: Patients in the standard therapy group were treated at the treating clinician's discretion following insertion of arterial and central venous catheterization, according to a protocol for hemodynamic support [target central venous pressure (CVP) 8–12 mm Hg, mean arterial pressure (MAP) ≥ 65 mm Hg, urine output ≥ 0.5 mL/kg/hr]. Antibiotics were given at the discretion of the treating clinician, and blood, urine, and other relevant specimens for culture were obtained prior to the administration of antibiotics.

Patients assigned to the EGDT group all received a central venous catheter (CVC) that was capable of measuring central venous oxygen saturation

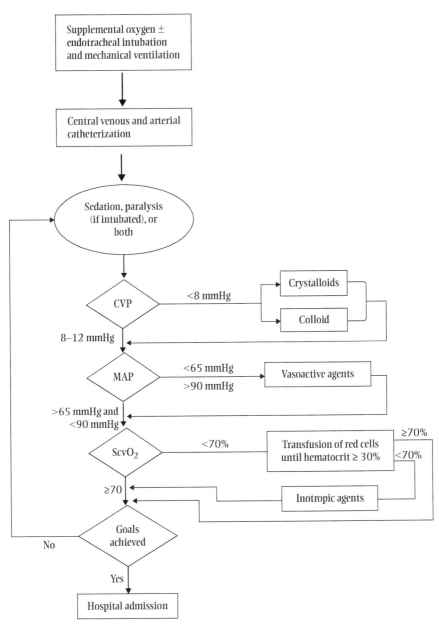

Figure 8.2 Protocol for Early Goal Directed Therapy. Reproduced with permission from Dr. E. Rivers.

($ScvO_2$) continuously or intermittently as performed in the control group. The control group was blinded to $ScvO_2$ and lactate results. Patients in this group were treated according to the EGDT protocol (Figure 8.2) in the ED for at least 6 hours prior to transfer to the first available intensive care inpatient bed, at which time monitoring of $ScvO_2$ was discontinued. The protocol for EGDT included a 500 mL bolus of crystalloid given every 30 minutes to achieve a CVP of 8–12 mm Hg, vasopressors to maintain a MAP of at least 65 mm Hg, and vasodilator use if MAP was greater than 90 mm Hg. If the $ScvO_2$ was less than 70% after fluid and vasopressor administration, then red cells were transfused to achieve a hematocrit of at least 30%. If the $ScvO_2$ remained less than 70% despite optimization of CVP, MAP, and hematocrit, then dobutamine was administered at a dose of 2.5 µg/kg of body weight per minute. This dose was increased by 2.5 µg/kg/min every 30 minutes until the $ScvO_2$ was 70% or higher or a maximum dose of 20 µg/kg/min was given. Dobutamine was decreased in dose or discontinued if the MAP was less than 65 mm Hg or if the heart rate was above 120 beats/min.

Follow-Up: 28 and 60 days or until death.

Endpoints: In-hospital mortality was the primary outcome measure. Secondary endpoint measurements included resuscitation endpoints, organ-dysfunction score, coagulation-related variables, administered treatments, and consumption of health care resources.

RESULTS

- During the first 6 hours, patients in the early goal-directed therapy group received more fluid, more blood transfusions, and more inotropic support than did patients in the standard-therapy group.
- During the first 6 hours, patients in the early goal-directed group had higher average MAPs and a higher average $ScvO_2$; in addition, a higher proportion achieved the combined goals for CVP, MAP, and urine output.
- During the period from 7 to 72 hours, patients in the early goal-directed therapy group had better hemodynamic parameters and required less fluid, red cell transfusions, vasopressors, and mechanical ventilation.
- Mortality was lower in the early goal-directed therapy group (see Table 8.1).

Table 8.1. KAPLAN-MEIR ESTIMATES OF MORTALITY AND CAUSES
OF IN-HOSPITAL DEATH

Variable	Standard therapy ($N = 133$)	EGDT therapy ($N = 130$)	Relative Risk (95% CI)	P Value
In-hospital mortality				
All patients	59 (46.5%)	38 (30.5%)	0.58 (0.38–0.87)	0.009
Patients with severe sepsis	19 (30.0%)	9 (14.9%)	0.46 (0.21–1.03)	0.06
Patients with septic shock	40 (56.8%)	29 (42.3%)	0.60 (0.36–0.98)	0.04
Patients with sepsis syndrome	44 (45.4%)	35 (35.1%)	0.66 (0.42–1.04)	0.07
28-Day mortality	61 (49.2%)	40 (33.3%)	0.58 (0.39–0.87)	0.01
60-Day mortality	70 (56.9%)	50 (44.3%)	0.67 (0.46–0.96)	0.03

Adapted from Rivers et al.

Criticisms and Limitations:

- This trial was conducted at a single center, so generalizability may be questioned.
- The study design does not reveal which components of EGDT were therapeutic or harmful, e.g., transfusion targets were higher, at what is now considered a more liberal transfusion strategy, during the study period and the EGDT group thus received larger volumes of transfusion in the first 6 hours of therapy.
- The trial was only partially blinded. In addition, there was potential for contamination of groups whereby as the study progressed, it is possible that patients in the standard therapy group received some components of EGDT and thus reduced the treatment effect.

Other Relevant Studies and Information:

- Since the publication of the EGDT trial, many observational and predominantly nonrandomized studies have supported the survival benefits seen in the original trial, even when there was incomplete implementation of the elements of the protocol.[2-5]
- Following the publication of the EGDT trial, there was widespread adoption of the concept of EGDT beginning with more aggressive sepsis identification and implementation of treatment algorithms with order sets.[6]

- The success of the EGDT trial was subsequently followed with trials of component therapies of the EGDT protocol, including use of central venous catheterization, transfusion strategies, vasopressor strategies, and systolic blood pressure targets.[7-13]
- Recently a trio of trials (ProCESS, ARISE, and ProMISe) questioned the continued need for all of the elements of early goal-directed therapy or the need for protocolized care for patients with severe sepsis and septic shock.[7-9] These trials were not direct replications of the original EGDT trial study design. Rather, they compared the current usual care to EGDT in patients with septic shock. While no mortality benefit was detected from EGDT in these trials, it is important to recognize that the results were obtained in the current era when standard care for sepsis has converged around the principles of early detection, early antibiotic therapy, and targeted fluid resuscitation as recommended by the Surviving Sepsis guidelines. This corresponds with a significant decline in mortality associated with septic shock from 46.5% in the EGDT trial[1] to 23.2% reported more recently.[2]
- The Surviving Sepsis Campaign (SSC) guidelines have incorporated elements of the EGDT trial, including immediate treatment and resuscitation, ongoing assessments of volume and tissue perfusion thorough clinical examination and evaluation of available physiologic variables, and use of noninvasive or invasive monitoring, as available.[16]
- The National Quality Forum (NQF) endorsed a measure for severe sepsis and septic shock that incorporates the fundamental concepts of EGDT.[14] It has been adopted as part of the first national quality measure for sepsis by the Centers for Medicare and Medicaid.

Summary and Implications: Publication of the EGDT trial shifted the paradigm of sepsis diagnosis and care from the ICU to the point of earliest presentation. Sepsis is now recognized for its occult nature, which may be unmasked by vigilance and laboratory assessment with lactate measurement. The utilization of EGDT at the earliest point of presentation has identified patients with the sepsis syndrome, severe sepsis, or septic shock, and has been endorsed by multiple societies including the SSC. Subsequent studies have raised questions about the value of individual components of the trial protocol, particularly the need for invasive central venous pressure monitoring upon initial presentation.

CLINICAL CASE: IMPLEMENTATION OF A SEPSIS GOAL-DIRECTED THERAPY BUNDLE IN THE ICU

Case History:

A 65-year-old male has been admitted to the ICU from the ED with septic shock. He had a lactate of 7 mmoL/L on initial assessment in the ED. He has received a total of 3000 mL of crystalloid solution prior to the ICU transfer and has an arterial line in place that shows a MAP of 63 mm Hg. Blood and urine cultures have been drawn and broad spectrum antibiotics have already been administered. How would you advise your junior resident to proceed in the management of this patient?

Suggested Answer:

The EGDT trial showed the greatest benefits in the patient population with an elevated lactate and low $ScvO_2$, indicative of a hemodynamic phenotype that is in the delivery-dependent phase of sepsis. EGDT is based on early identification of high-risk patients with incorporation of lactate measurement for risk stratification followed by antibiotic administration, source control, and hemodynamic support.

This patient with septic shock has already received 30 cc/kg of crystalloid fluid but should be further assessed for a state of continued fluid responsiveness. For each intervention that is performed, assessment and re-assessment of the patient is mandatory and may be assessed with lactate clearance, along with monitoring the constellation of resuscitative markers. If the MAP remains <65 mm Hg without signs of hypovolemia, vasoactive agents are preferred for a target goal of ≥ 65 mm Hg. A CVC can be placed for central administration of vasoactive agents, and it also provides the added benefit of additional hemodynamic measurements, including CVP and $ScvO_2$. Elements of the EGDT protocol are targeted toward the delivery-dependent phase, and vigilance is necessary to address transitions to delivery-independent phases of sepsis and identification of recovery when therapies may need to be reduced or escalated.

References

1. Rivers E, Nguyen B, Havstad S et al. Early Goal-Directed Therapy Collaborative Group. Early goal-directed therapy in the treatment of severe sepsis and septic shock. *N Engl J Med*. 2001;345(19):1368–1377.
2. Angus DC, Barnato AE, Bell D et al. A systematic review and meta-analysis of early goal-directed therapy for septic shock: the ARISE, ProCESS and ProMISe Investigators. *Intensive Care Med*. 2015;41(9):1549–1560.
3. Coba V, Whitmill M, Mooney R et al. Resuscitation bundle compliance in severe sepsis and septic shock: improves survival, is better late than never. *J Intensive Care Med*. 2011;26(5):304–313.
4. Huang DT, Clermont G, Dremsizov TT, Angus DC; ProCESS Investigators. Implementation of early goal-directed therapy for severe sepsis and septic shock: A decision analysis. *Crit Care Med*. 2007;35(9):2090–2100.
5. Jones AE, F.A., Horton JM, Kline JA. Prospective external validation of the clinical effectiveness of an emergency department-based early goal-directed therapy protocol for severe sepsis and septic shock. *Chest*. 2007;132(2):425–432.

6. Whippy A, Skeath M, Crawford B et al. Permanente's performance improvement system, part 3: multisite improvements in care for patients with sepsis. *Jt Comm J Qual Patient Saf.* 2011;37(11):483–493.

7. ProCESS Investigators, Yealy DM, Kellum JA, Huang DT, et al. A randomized trial of protocol-based care for early septic shock. *N Engl J Med.* 2014;370(18):1683–1693.

8. ARISE Investigators; ANZICS Clinical Trials Group, Peake SL, Delaney A, Bailey M, et al. Goal-directed resuscitation for patients with early septic shock. *N Engl J Med.* 2014;371(16):1496–1506.

9. Mouncey PR, Osborn TM, Power GS et al. Trial of early, goal-directed resusctiation for septic shock. *N Engl J Med.* 2015. 372(14):1301–1311.

10. Holst LB, Haase N, Wetterslev J et al. TRISS trial group; Scandinavian Critical Care Trials Group. Lower versus higher hemoglobin threshold for transfusion in septic shock. *N Engl J Med.* 2014;371(15):1381–1391.

11. Russell JA, Walley KR, Singer J, et al. VASST Investigators. Vasopressin versus norepinephrine infusion in patients with septic shock. *N Engl J Med.* 2008;358(9): 877–887.

12. De Backer D1, Biston P, Devriendt J, et al. SOAP II Investigators. Comparison of dopamine and norepinephrine in the treatment of shock. *N Engl J Med.* 2010;362(9):779–789.

13. Asfar P, Meziani F, Hamel JF et al. *High versus low blood-pressure target in patients with septic shock.* N Engl J Med, 2014. 370(17): 1583–1593.

14. National Quality Forum. Severe Sepsis and Septic Shock: Management Bundle (NQF 0500). Washington, DC: National Quality Forum; 2015. Available at: http://emcrit.org/wp-content/uploads/2015/06/0500.pd

15. Nguyen HB, Jaehne AK, Jayaprakash N et al. Early goal-directed therapy in severe sepsis and septic shock: insights and comparisons to ProCESS, ProMISe, and ARISE. *Crit Care,* 2016; 20(1): 1–16.

16. Shankar-Hari M, Phillips GS, Levy ML, et al. Developing a new definition and assessing new clinical criteria for septic shock: For the third international consensus definitions for sepsis and septic shock (sepsis-3). *JAMA,* 2016. 315(8): 775–787.

Lactate Clearance versus Central Venous Oxygen Saturation as Goals of Early Sepsis Therapy

MARC DE MOYA AND LEANDRA KROWSOSKI

"The results of this large multicenter randomized controlled trial of 2 resuscitation protocols for early sepsis resuscitation indicate that a protocol targeting lactate clearance of at least 10% as evidence of adequate tissue oxygen delivery produces a similar short-term survival rate as a protocol using ScvO$_2$ [central venous oxygen saturation] monitoring."
—THE EMERGENCY MEDICINE SHOCK RESEARCH
NETWORK INVESTIGATORS

Research Question: Is in-house mortality equivalent when using lactate clearance as a goal of early sepsis resuscitation as compared to using central venous oxygen saturation (ScvO$_2$) monitoring as recommended by the Surviving Sepsis Campaign guidelines?[1,2]

Funding: National Institutes of Health (NIH), National Institute of General Medical Sciences

Year Study Began: 2007

Year Study Published: 2010

Study Location: 3 large urban US hospitals

Who Was Studied: Patients older than 17 years old presenting to the emergency department with evidence of infection, meeting at least 2 criteria for systemic inflammatory response syndrome,[3] and with evidence of hypoperfusion (systolic blood pressure < 90 mm Hg despite a fluid bolus or elevated lactate concentration > 36 mg/dL or 4 mmol/L).

Who Was Excluded: Patients who were pregnant, had a primary diagnosis other than sepsis, might require surgery within 6 hours of diagnosis, had contraindications to chest or neck central venous catheters, required cardiopulmonary resuscitation, were transferred from another institution with a sepsis resuscitation protocol initiated, or with advanced directives preventing interventions required by the study protocol were excluded.

How Many Patients: A total of 300 patients were randomized.

Study Overview: The study was designed to determine the non-inferiority of lactate clearance as a marker of adequate oxygen delivery compared to $ScvO_2$. Each group underwent a parallel targeted resuscitative protocol in the emergency department, including targeted central venous pressure (CVP) and mean arterial pressure (MAP) goals. The study design is summarized in Figure 9.1.

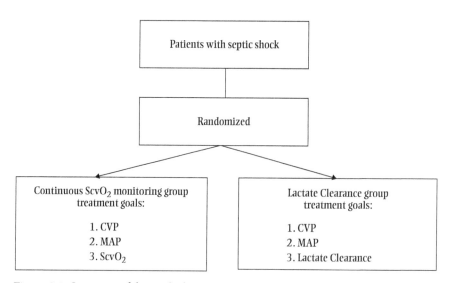

Figure 9.1 Summary of the study design.

Study Intervention: Chest or neck central venous catheters were placed in all patients. The central venous catheters of patients in the $ScvO_2$ group were connected to continuous monitoring.

The protocol for the ScvO$_2$ group was carried out in the following order:
1. Isotonic crystalloid boluses were given until a CVP ≥ to 8 mm Hg was reached.
2. If the MAP was < 65 mm Hg after the goal CVP was reached, then dopamine or norepinephrine were initiated and titrated to the MAP goal.
3. After CVP and MAP goals were achieved, if ScvO$_2$ was < 70% and the hematocrit < 30%, packed red blood cells were transfused to a hematocrit of 30%. If ScvO$_2$ was less than 70% after the appropriate transfusion, then dobutamine was started and titrated for the ScvO$_2$ goal.

The protocol for the lactate clearance group provided identical interventions to achieve the targeted CVP and MAP goals; however a lactate clearance goal of 10% was substituted as the tertiary goal. This study defined lactate clearance as

$$\left[\left(\text{lactate}_{\text{initial}} - \text{lactate}_{\text{delayed}}\right)/\text{lactate}_{\text{initial}}\right] \times 100\%$$

Lactate$_{\text{initial}}$ was measured at the start of resuscitation and lactate$_{\text{delayed}}$ was measured 2 hours later. If the lactate clearance was < 10% after the first two hour measurement and the hematocrit was < 30%, packed red blood cells were transfused to achieve the hematocrit threshold. If the hematocrit was ≥ 30%, dobutamine was started and titrated. Lactate measurements were continued at 1 hour intervals thereafter until a lactate clearance of 10% was achieved (or if both initial and delayed lactate concentrations were not elevated).

Study interventions were performed in the emergency department from the time of randomization until all treatment goals were achieved or until 6 hours had elapsed.

Follow-Up: Data collection continued for 72 hours post transfer from the emergency department to the ICU, then daily follow-up continued until hospital discharge or death.

Endpoints: Absolute in-hospital mortality was the primary endpoint. ICU length of stay, hospital length of stay, ventilator-free days and new-onset multiple organ failure were secondary endpoints.

RESULTS

- 29 patients (10%) required dobutamine infusion or packed red blood cell transfusion in the initial resuscitation period to meet lactate clearance or ScvO$_2$ goals.
- In-hospital mortality rate was 17% in the lactate clearance group versus 23% in the SvcO$_2$ group in intent-to-treat analysis.

- Non-inferiority was confirmed: the confidence interval of the difference in mortality rates was above the established threshold of -10.
- Length of ICU stay was 5.9 days in the lactate clearance group versus 5.6 days in the ScvO$_2$ group. Length of hospital stay was 11.4 days in the lactate clearance group versus 12.1 days in the ScvO$_2$ group.
- The mean number of ventilator free days in the lactate clearance group was 9.3 days versus 9.9 days in the ScvO$_2$ group.
- Multiple organ failure occurred in 25% of patients in the lactate clearance group and 22% of patients in the ScvO$_2$ group (Table 9.1).

Table 9.1. SUMMARY OF THE STUDY'S KEY FINDINGS

End point	Lactate Clearance Group ($n = 1500$)	ScvO$_2$ Group ($n = 150$)	Proportion Difference (95% Confidence Interval)	P-value
In-hospital mortality	25 (17%)	34 (23%)	6 (-3 to 15)	
Mean length of ICU stay, days	5.9	5.6		0.75
Mean length of hospital stay, days	11.4	12.1		0.64
Mean ventilator-free days	9.3	9.9		0.67
Multiple organ failure	37 (25%)	33 (22%)		0.68

Criticisms and Limitations:

- The groups in the study were not blinded, which could result in treatment bias; granted blinding was impossible given the nature of the study.
- In addition, the three hospitals involved in the study had formal emergency department sepsis resuscitation protocols in place. Therefore results may not be generalizable to institutions without such programs.
- Because only 10% of patients in the study required the intervention of dobutamine or packed red blood cell transfusion, the impact that lactate clearance versus ScvO$_2$ had on the endpoints of the study is potentially small.
- Finally, knowing that the study was in progress may have led clinicians to be more attentive in their overall care of patients and led to an effect on survival and the other endpoints.

Other Relevant Studies and Information:

- Use of lactate clearance as a representative of tissue perfusion was based on the presumption that shock causes tissue hypoxia leading to utilization of anaerobic glycolysis and production of lactate as a byproduct of metabolism.[4]

- Additional studies have shown that lactate clearance of 10% or more in sepsis resuscitation predicts survival.[5,6,7]
- Practically, lack of familiarity with $ScvO_2$ measurement and interpretation requires training of staff and can impact workflow in the emergency department during the initial resuscitation period.[8]

Summary and Implications: $ScvO_2$ measured via central venous catheter has been established as a marker of tissue perfusion in resuscitation for sepsis. The results of this study show that lactate clearance can be used in place of $ScvO_2$ as part of a resuscitation protocol that includes quantitative goals for CVP and MAP to yield an equivalent short-term survival outcome.

CLINICAL CASE: LACTATE CLEARANCE VERSUS CENTRAL VENOUS OXYGEN SATURATION

Case History:
A 60-year-old woman presents to the emergency department with fever, a systolic blood pressure of 85 unresponsive to a fluid bolus, and a chest x-ray consistent with right lower lobe pneumonia. Prior to her transfer to the ICU, you plan on initiating early goal directed therapy for sepsis. Based on the results of the Lactate Clearance versus Central Venous Oxygen Saturation study, should you continuously monitor $ScvO_2$ as part of her emergency department resuscitation?

Suggested Answer:
This study showed that the use of lactate clearance instead of $ScvO_2$ as part of a resuscitation bundle results in equivalent in-hospital mortality. Either measuring lactate clearance or $ScvO_2$ as a tertiary goal of early sepsis resuscitation after achieving a goal CVP and MAP is reasonable. Other practical factors, such as staff comfort with $ScvO_2$ monitoring, should then be considered when deciding which marker of tissue perfusion to trend.

References

1. Jones AE, Shapiro NI, Trzeciak S, Arnold RC, Claremont HA, Kline JA. Lactate Clearance vs Central Venous Oxygen Saturation as Goals of Early Sepsis Therapy: A Randomized Clinical Trial. *JAMA.* 2010;303(8):739–746.
2. Rivers E, Nguyen B, Havstad S, et al., Early Goal-Directed Therapy Collaborative Group. Early goal-directed therapy in the treatment of severe sepsis and septic shock. *N Engl J Med.* 2001;345(19):1368–1377.

3. Bone RC, Balk RA, Cerra FB, et al., The ACCP/SCCM Consensus Conference Committee. American College of Chest Physicians/Society of Critical Care Medicine. Definitions for sepsis and organ failure and guidelines for the use of innovative therapies in sepsis. *Chest.* 1992;101(6):1644–1655.
4. Watts JA, Kline JA. Bench to bedside: the role of mitochondrial medicine in the pathogenesis and treatment of cellular injury. *Acad Emerg Med.* 2003;10(9):985–997.
5. Arnold RC, Shapiro NI, Jones AE, et al. Multicenter study of early lactate clearance as a determinant of survival in patients with presumed sepsis. *Shock.* 2009;32(1):35–39.
6. Walker CA, Griffith DM, Gray AJ, Datta D, Hay AW. Early lactate clearance in septic patients with elevated lactate levels admitted from the emergency department to intensive care: time to aim higher? *J Crit Care.* 2013;28(5):832–837.
7. Marty P, Roquilly A, Vallée F, et al. Lactate clearance for death prediction in severe sepsis or septic shock patients during the first 24 hours in Intensive Care Unit: an observational study. *Ann Intensive Care.* 2013;3(1):3.
8. Jones AE, Shapiro NI, Roshon M. Implementing early goal-directed therapy in the emergency setting: the challenges and experiences of translating research innovations into clinical reality in academic and community settings. *Acad Emerg Med.* 2007;14(11):1072–1078.

Efficacy and Safety of Recombinant Human Activated Protein C for Severe Sepsis

The PROWESS Study

ANNA M. WARD AND RICHARD M. PINO

"The administration of drotrecogin alfa activated reduced the rate of death from any cause at 28 days in patients with a clinical diagnosis of severe sepsis resulting in a 19.4% reduction in the relative risk of death and an absolute reduction of 6.1%. Our results indicate that in this population, 1 additional life would be saved for every 16 patients treated with drotrecogin alfa activated."

—BERNARD ET AL.

Research Question: Drotrecogin alfa (activated) (DAA) is a recombinant form of human activated protein C that has antithrombotic, anti-inflammatory, and profibrinolytic properties. It has been shown to produce dose-dependent reductions in markers of inflammation in patients with severe sepsis. Does treatment with DAA reduce the rate of death from any cause among patients with severe sepsis?[1]

Sponsor: Eli Lilly and Company

Year Study Began: July 1998

Year Study Published: 2001

Study Location: 164 centers in 11 countries

Who Was Studied: Patients with known or suspected infection on the basis of clinical data at the time of screening who had three or more signs of systemic inflammation and sepsis-induced dysfunction of at least one organ or system in a 24 hour period. Treatment began within 24 hours of meeting the inclusion criteria. Three-fourths of patients enrolled in both placebo and treatment groups had at least two dysfunctional organs or systems with the abdomen and lungs as the most common sites of infection.

Who Was Excluded: Exclusions included patients with coexisting illnesses with a high risk of death (i.e., metastatic cancer), an increased risk of bleeding (i.e., acute pancreatitis), an increased risk of thrombosis secondary to a hypercoagulable state, recent treatment with anti-thrombolytic agents, and those with major chronic illnesses such as renal failure requiring dialysis, and cirrhosis.

How Many Patients: 1728 patients underwent randomization and 1690 received the study drug or placebo.

Study Overview: This phase III, randomized, double-blind, placebo-controlled, multicenter trial was designed to evaluate whether treatment with DAA would reduce the rate of death from all causes at 28 days in patients with systemic inflammation and organ failure due to acute infection (Figure 10.1).

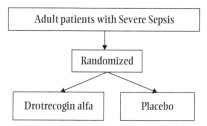

Figure 10.1 Overall cumulative mortality rate for the PROWESS trial. Figure B: Cumulative mortality rate for sites enrolling patients under both the original and amended protocol. (Reproduced with permission from Macias M, et al.,*Critical Care Medicine* 2004;32(12):2385–2391.)

Study Intervention: Patients were randomly assigned to receive an intravenous dose of DAA at a dose of 24 mcg/kg/hr or placebo (0.9% saline with or without 0.1% human serum albumin) for 96 hours within 24 hours of meeting inclusion criteria. Infusions were interrupted 1 hour before any percutaneous procedure or major surgery and were resumed 1 hour and 12 hours later, respectively. The study protocol had no standardized approach to critical care treatment such as the use of antibiotics, fluids, vasopressors, or respiratory support with both groups receiving standard supportive care.

Follow-Up: Patients were followed for 28 days after the start of the infusion or until death.

Endpoints: The primary endpoint was death from any cause and was assessed 28 days after the initiation of the infusion. No secondary endpoints were specified.

RESULTS

- Baseline characteristics were similar in the treatment and placebo groups including age (mean 60), sex (58% male), race (82% white), APACHE II scores (25), and prior or preexisting medical conditions.
- Protein C deficiency (as defined as levels below the lower limit of normal 81%) was present in 87.6% of patients (Table 10.1).

Table 10.1. ANALYSIS OF THE RATES AND RISKS OF DEATH FROM ANY CAUSE AT 28 DAYS. IN THE PROSPECTIVELY DEFINED STRATIFIED ANALYSIS (PRESENCE OR ABSENCE OF PROTEIN C DEFICIENCY) THE RELATIVE RISK OF DEATH WAS CALCULATED AFTER AN ADJUSTMENT FOR THE BASELINE APACHE II SCORE, AGE, AND PROTEIN C ACTIVITY

	Placebo Group	Drotrecogin Alfa Activated Group	P Value	Relative Risk of Death (95% CI)	Absolute Risk Reduction (95% CI)
Nonstratified analysis	259/840 (31%)	210/850 (25%)	0.005	0.80 (0.69 to 0.94)	6.1 (1.9 to 10.4)
Protein C deficiency					
Yes	215/670 (32%)	182/709 (26%)	0.009	0.80 (0.68 to 0.95)	6.4 (1.6 to 11.2)
No	28/105 (27%)	14/90 (16%)	0.06	0.58 (0.33 to 1.04)	11.1 (−0.4 to 22.6)
Unknown	16/65 (25%)	14/51 (27%)	0.73	1.12 (0.60 to 2.07)	−2.8 (−19.0 to 13.4)

- At 28 days after the start of the infusion, 259 of 840 patients in the placebo group (31%) and 210 of 850 (25%) in the DAA group died. The difference in the rate of death from any cause was statistically significant ($P = 0.005$) and associated with a 6.1% absolute reduction in the risk of death.

- Plasma D-dimer and interleukin-6 levels were lower in patients in the DAA group than the placebo group 1–7 days after starting the infusion. There was no difference in the effect of treatment with DAA among the subgroup with known protein C deficiency and those with normal protein C levels.
- The incidence of serious bleeding was higher in the DAA (3.5%) versus the placebo (2%) group. Fatal intracranial hemorrhages were found in two of the DAA treated patients during the infusion (day 1 and day 4) and one in the placebo group six days after the end of the infusion. Blood transfusion requirements were the same in both groups.

Criticisms and Limitations:

- The PROWESS trial relied on patients enrolled in 164 international centers with varied practice patterns, heterogeneous patient populations with gradations in severity of illness, and underlying infectious etiologies and chronic medical conditions. Interpretation of results is confounded by this variability in addition to differences in what is considered the standard of care in treatment for patients with severe sepsis at the variety of centers participating in the trial. However, because the trial was randomized, the impact of these confounding factors on trial results is likely to be modest.
- The study protocol was amended to clarify the intent in the original version to exclude patients who were likely to die from underlying non-sepsis related medical conditions within the 28-day study period and to also allow the introduction of a new form of DAA produced from a new master cell bank derived from the original cell bank.[2,3] About 760 patients were enrolled under the original version of the protocol with the remainder under the amended version. The observed treatment effect appeared to be larger for patients enrolled under the amended protocol. Mortality in the DAA treatment group progressively decreased throughout the study whereas the placebo mortality rate appeared to be relatively stable (Figure 10.1).[3] Patient characteristics between those enrolled under the original protocol versus the amended protocol were not statistically different.
- Subsequent subgroup analyses of the PROWESS trial data suggested that decreased absolute difference in mortality, but not relative risk of death, was most notable in patients with greater illness severity as measured by Acute Physiology and Chronic Health Evaluation (APACHE) II score >24 (on a scale of 0 to 71, with higher scores

indicating an increased risk of death) or the number of dysfunctional organs at the onset of severe sepsis.[4] There was no apparent benefit in subjects at lower risk of death (lower APACHE II score) or those with single organ dysfunction but the number of events (deaths) in these groups was also very low, thus limiting the statistical power to detect a difference if there was one.

Other Relevant Studies and Information:

- The initial publication of the PROWESS trial was met with great enthusiasm. In November 2001, the FDA expedited the approval for the use of DAA for patients with severe sepsis at high risk of death as determined by a high APACHE II score. However, this enthusiasm waned over time as the data was subject to further subgroup analysis and in light of the apparent mortality benefit occurring after the protocol was amended halfway through the trial. In its review, the FDA recommended conducting additional pediatric and adult multi-center, placebo controlled trials to further characterize the effects of DAA in children and in adults with severe sepsis but with low APACHE scores.[2] These subsequent studies are discussed as follows:

- Administration of Drotrecogin Alfa Activated in Early Stage Severe Sepsis (ADDRESS trial). A randomized double-blind, placebo-controlled study evaluating the efficacy of DAA in patients with severe sepsis at lower risk of death (APACHE II score < 25 or single organ dysfunction) was completed in 2005 and found no statistical difference in 28-day mortality (17% placebo versus 18.5% DAA, $P = 0.34$). The trial found an increased risk of serious bleeding with DAA (2.4%) compared to placebo (1.2%).[5]

- Researching Severe Sepsis and Organ Dysfunction in Children (RESOLVE trial). In this study published in 2005, 240 children with sepsis-induced cardiovascular and respiratory failure received DAA and 237 received placebo. Mortality at 28 days was not improved (17.5% placebo versus 17.7% DAA, $P = 0.39$). The risk of bleeding was equal between placebo and activated protein C groups, except in children less than 60 days old.[6]

- Drotrecogin Alfa (Activated) in Adults with Septic Shock (PROWESS-SHOCK). The randomized, double-blind, placebo-controlled, multicenter trial started in 2008 and published in 2011 was a follow-up to the original PROWESS. Similar to the original PROWESS study, 1,696 patients with septic shock were randomized to receive either placebo or DAA at a dose of 24 mcg/kg/hr for 96 hours. This study found no difference in mortality in patients with severe sepsis who were treated with DAA versus those who received placebo.[7] In October 2011 following the failure of the PROWESS-SHOCK trial to confirm the mortality benefit of DAA in septic patients that was reported in the original PROWESS trial, Eli Lilly and Company voluntarily withdrew the drug from the market.[8]

Summary and Implications: The PROWESS trial demonstrated a mortality benefit for DAA among patients with severe sepsis. However, the subsequent ADDRESS, RESOLVE, and PROWESS-SHOCK trials did not demonstrate a benefit of the medication, thus calling the results of PROWESS into question. The initial decision by the FDA to approve DAA on the basis of this single phase III trial (PROWESS) demonstrates the potential danger in widespread adoption of new therapeutics without first obtaining sufficient data on benefits and risks. Indeed, most drugs approved for use in the United States are based on at least two positive phase III trials demonstrating clinical efficacy.

CLINICAL CASE: EFFICACY AND SAFETY OF RECOMBINANT HUMAN ACTIVATED PROTEIN C FOR SEVERE SEPSIS

Case History:
A 54-year-old woman with Type 2 diabetes mellitus was admitted to the ICU with a 3-day history of nausea, vomiting, fever, chills, and flank pain in June 2009. Her husband stated she had been complaining of mild dysuria and increased urinary frequency. She received 1.5 liters of crystalloid in the ED before being transferred to the ICU. On arrival to the ICU, her vital signs were as follows: blood pressure 75/40 mm Hg, heart rate 127 bpm, respiratory rate 18 bpm, temperature 102.8°F. Her labs were significant for a lactate of 2.9 mmol/L. In addition to the standard of care for the treatment of sepsis, the patient was started on an infusion of DAA and 24 hours of admission to the ICU. Five days later, she was transferred out of the ICU in stable condition. Did the administration of DAA result in the resolution of her sepsis?

Suggested Answer:
DAA was withdrawn from the market after this patient's illness. Given the lack of evidence to support the efficacy of DAA in the treatment of patients with sepsis, she would have probably not benefited from its administration. DAA would also have increased her risk of bleeding from any cause during its infusion.

References

1. Bernard GR, Vincent JL, Laterre PF, et al. Efficacy and safety of recombinant human activated protein C for severe sepsis. *New Engl J Med*. 2001;344:699–709.
2. Finfer S, Ranieri VM, Thompson BT, et al. Design, conduct, analysis and reporting of a multi-national placebo-controlled trial of activated protein C for persistent septic shock. *Intensive Care Med*. 2008;34(11):1935–1947.
3. Macias WL, Vallet B, Bernard GR, et al. Sources of variability on the estimate of treatment effect in the PROWESS trial: Implications for the design and conduct of future studies in severe sepsis. *Crit Care Med*. 2004;32(12):2385–2391.
4. Ely EW, Laterre PF, Angus DC, et al. Drotrecogin alfa (activated) administration across clinically important subgroups of patients with severe sepsis. *Crit Care Med*. 2003;31:12–19.
5. Abraham E, Laterre PF, Garg R, et al. Drotrecogin alfa (activated) for adults with severe sepsis and a low risk of death. *New Engl J Med*. 2005;353:1332–1341.
6. Nadel S, Goldsetin B, Williams MD, et al. Drotrecogin alfa (activated) in children with severe sepsis: a multicenter phase III randomized controlled trial. *Lancet*. 2007;369:836–843.
7. Ranieri VM, Thompson BT, Barie PS, et al. Drotrecogin alfa (activated) in adults with septic shock. *New Engl J Med*. 2012;366(22):2055–2064.
8. Friedrich JO, Adhikari N, Meade OM. Drotrecogin alfa (activated): does current evidence support treatment for any patients with severe sepsis? *Crit Care*. 2006;10(145).

11

Saline versus Albumin for Resuscitation of Critically Ill Adults

The SAFE Study

CRAIG S. JABALEY

> "Our study provides evidence that albumin and saline should be considered clinically equivalent treatments for intravascular volume resuscitation in . . . the ICU."
>
> —THE SAFE STUDY INVESTIGATORS

Research Question: Does the administration of albumin compared with saline for fluid resuscitation have an impact on the mortality of critically ill patients?[1]

Sponsors: Multiple research councils, government agency grants, and hospitals in Australia and New Zealand.[2]

Year Study Began: 2001

Year Study Published: 2004

Study Location: Multidisciplinary closed intensive care units (ICUs) of 16 academic tertiary hospitals in Australia and New Zealand.

Who Was Studied: Patients 18 years of age or older admitted to an ICU for whom the treating clinician judged that fluid administration was required to maintain or increase intravascular volume, with this decision supported by the fulfillment of at least one objective criterion (see Box 11.1).

BOX 11.1. INCLUSION CRITERIA USED TO SUPPORT THE NEED FOR FLUID RESUSCITATION. AT LEAST ONE CRITERION WAS REQUIRED.

- Heart Rate > 90
- Systolic blood pressure < 100 mm Hg
- Mean arterial pressure < 75 mm Hg
- Decrease in baseline systolic or mean blood pressure ≥ 40 mm Hg
- Requirement of vasopressors or inotropes to maintain blood pressure
- Central venous pressure < 10 mm Hg
- Pulmonary capillary wedge pressure < 12 mm Hg
- Respiratory variation in systolic or mean arterial blood pressure > 5 mm Hg
- Capillary refill time > 1 second
- Urine output < 0.5 mL/kg for 1 hour

Who Was Excluded: Patients admitted to an ICU after cardiac surgery, liver transplantation, or having sustained burns were excluded.

How Many Patients: 6997

Study Overview: See Figure 11.1 for an overview of the study design.

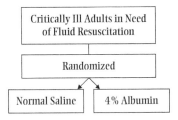

Figure 11.1 Summary of the study design.

Study Intervention: After enrollment in the trial, patients were randomized to receive either albumin or normal saline whenever intravascular volume expansion was deemed necessary by the treating clinician for the duration of the patient's ICU stay. The volume, rate, and timing of study fluid administration were all left at the discretion of the treating clinician. Concealment was accomplished with cartons to mask study fluid vials and paired opaque administration sets. Study fluids were administered in addition to routine maintenance or replacement fluids, enteral or parenteral nutrition, and/or blood products as also directed by the treating clinician.

Follow-Up: 28 days after randomization

Endpoints: All-cause 28-day mortality was the primary outcome measure. Secondary measures included survival time, sequential organ-failure assessment (SOFA) score, duration of mechanical ventilation, duration of renal replacement therapy, ICU length of stay (LOS), and hospital LOS. Death from any cause within 28 days after randomization was also examined in three predefined subgroups: trauma, sepsis, and acute respiratory distress syndrome at baseline.

RESULTS

- The average ratio of albumin to saline administered to patients during the first four days of the study was 1:1.4. Mean arterial pressure at the end of each of the first four days did not differ significantly between the two groups. Patients in the albumin group received a greater volume of packed red blood cells during study days one and two.
- There was no difference in 28-day all-cause mortality between the albumin (20.9%) and saline (21.1%) groups (95% CI 0.91–1.09, $P = 0.87$).
- There were no significant differences in ICU or hospital LOS, duration of mechanical ventilation, duration of renal replacement therapy, or the incidence of organ failure.
- Analysis of the three predefined subgroups revealed a heightened relative risk of death in the albumin group among trauma patients. This increased mortality was most pronounced in the subset of patients with traumatic brain injury (TBI) who received albumin, where the relative risk of death was 1.62 (95% CI 1.12–2.34, $P = 0.009$). Among trauma patients without TBI, the relative risk of death was not significant.
- There was a non-significant trend toward reduced mortality among patients with sepsis who were resuscitated with albumin (RR 0.87, 95% CI 0.74–1.02, $P = 0.09$).

Criticisms and Limitations:

- The study lacked sufficient power to detect differences in mortality among the predefined subgroups.

- Death at 28 days may not be the most appropriate outcome measure for patients with brain injury. Assessment of ICP elevation, need for treatment, or functional outcomes may have been more appropriate.
- It has been suggested that patients in the study were not markedly hypovolemic as baseline central venous pressures were about 9 mm Hg in both groups and increased to only 11 mm Hg (in the albumin group) and 10 mm Hg (in the saline group) during the four days of the study. Furthermore, the baseline heart rates and mean arterial pressures, as well as responses to the infusions, do not suggest severe hypovolemia. It is possible that the results would have been different in a more hypovolemic patient population.

Other Relevant Studies and Information:

- A follow-up study of patients with TBI that were enrolled in the SAFE trial examined mortality and neurologic outcomes at 24 months.[3] Patients with TBI that received albumin were found to have an increased relative risk of death at 24 months of 1.63 (95% CI 1.17–2.26, P = 0.003). When stratified by severity of TBI, those with severe TBI (GCS 3-8) demonstrated a significantly increased relative risk of death (RR 1.88, 95% CI 1.13–2.70, P < 0.001), the majority of which was within the first 28 days. In comparison, no statistically significant difference was observed for those with moderate TBI (GCS 9–12).
- Another post-hoc study of patients with severe sepsis that were enrolled in the SAFE trial suggested that albumin resuscitation may be beneficial in patients with severe sepsis.[4] Using multivariate logistic regression to control for confounders, the study found an odds ratio for mortality of 0.71 (95% CI 0.52–0.97, P = 0.03) when compared with saline.
- The 2014 ALBIOS study further investigated the use of albumin administration to maintain the serum albumin level ≥30 g/L in patients with severe sepsis or septic shock.[5] While there was no difference in survival at 28 and 90 days, those treated with albumin had more favorable SOFA subscores and received fewer vasopressors or inotropes. Post-hoc subgroup multivariate analysis suggested that patients with septic shock may benefit from albumin replacement.
- A 2013 Cochrane review found no benefit of albumin over crystalloids for fluid resuscitation in critically ill patients (all-cause mortality RR 1.01; 95% CI 0.93–1.10), leading the authors to

conclude that the use of colloids is unjustified given their increased cost and lack of benefit.[6]

• The Surviving Sepsis Campaign guidelines (2016) suggest using albumin in addition to crystalloids for resuscitation in patients with sepsis and septic shock when patients require substantial amounts of crystalloids (grade 2C).[7]

Summary and Implications: The study provides evidence that albumin and saline can be considered clinically equivalent treatments for fluid resuscitation in a heterogeneous population of critically ill patients. Because of its lower cost, saline is considered the preferred fluid for resuscitation, except perhaps among patients with severe sepsis requiring considerable amounts of crystalloid.

CLINICAL CASE: RESUSCITATION FLUID CHOICE IN THE ICU

Case History:

A 65-year-old female is admitted to the ICU with septic shock owing to suspected pneumonia. Fluid resuscitation was begun in the emergency department. Based on the results of this study, should the patient receive crystalloids or albumin for further resuscitation?

Suggested Answer:

The SAFE study suggests that albumin and saline should be considered clinically equivalent treatments for fluid resuscitation in critically ill patients (without TBI). Although some critical care physicians consider albumin administration after extensive crystalloid resuscitation in an effort to reduce the likelihood of volume overload, this practice is not well-supported by the available literature. While exploratory findings suggest that albumin may be beneficial in patients with severe sepsis and septic shock, the available evidence does not support its use as the primary resuscitation fluid used in the care of this patient.

References

1. The SAFE Study investigators. a comparison of albumin and saline for fluid resuscitation in the intensive care unit. *N Engl J Med.* 2004;350(22):2247–2256.
2. ANZICS Clinical Trials Group, SAFE Study Investigators. The Saline vs. Albumin Fluid Evaluation (SAFE) Study (ISRCTN76588266): Design and conduct of a multicentre, blinded randomised controlled trial of intravenous fluid resuscitation in critically ill patients. *BMJ.* 2004;326(7389):559–560, Online Suppl.

3. The SAFE Study Investigators. Saline or albumin for fluid resuscitation in patients with traumatic brain injury. *N Engl J Med.* 2007;357(9):874–884.

4. The SAFE Study Investigators. Impact of albumin compared to saline on organ function and mortality of patients with severe sepsis. *Intensive Care Med.* 2010;37(1):86–96.

5. Caironi P, Tognoni G, Masson S, et al. Albumin replacement in patients with severe sepsis or septic shock. *N Engl J Med.* 2014;370(15):1412–1421.

6. Perel P, Roberts I, Ker K. Colloids versus crystalloids for fluid resuscitation in critically ill patients. *Cochrane Database Syst Rev.* 2013:CD000567. DOI: 10.1002/14651858. CD000567.pub6.

7. Rhodes A, Evans LE, Alhazzani W, et al. Surviving sepsis campaign: international guidelines for management of sepsis and septic shock: 2016. *Crit Care Med.* 2017;45(3):486–552.

12

The Use of the Pulmonary Artery Catheter in Critical Care

The PAC-Man Trial

SHAHZAD SHAEFI AND AMEEKA PANNU

"Our results indicate no difference in hospital mortality between critically ill patients managed with or without a PAC."
—THE PAC-MAN INVESTIGATORS

Research Question: Is hospital mortality reduced in critically ill patients with the use of a pulmonary artery catheter (PAC)?[1]

Funding: UK NHS Research and Development Health Technology Assessment Programme

Year Study Began: 2001

Year Study Published: 2005

Study Location: 65 ICUs in the United Kingdom

Who Was Studied: Patients admitted to adult intensive care in the United Kingdom and identified by the treating clinician as someone who should be managed with a PAC

Who Was Excluded: (1) Patients younger than 16 years, (2) patients admitted electively to the ICU for preoperative optimization, (3) patients who had a PAC on admission to the ICU, (4) patients previously enrolled in the study, (5) patients undergoing hemodynamic optimization before organ donation

How Many Patients: 1263 eligible, 1041 enrolled

Study Overview: This was a prospective randomized controlled trial examining the *effectiveness* rather than the *efficacy* of the use of PAC. Patients enrolled in the study were admitted to an adult intensive care unit in the United Kingdom and identified by the treating physician as someone who should be managed with a pulmonary artery catheter (PAC). Patients were then randomized by a central 24-hour telephone service and assigned to one of two groups: management with or without a PAC. The minimization for randomization was based on age, presumptive clinical status, and surgical status (Figure 12.1).

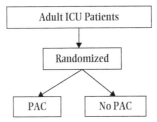

Figure 12.1 Summary of the study design.

Study Intervention: In patients allocated to the PAC group, a PAC was placed as soon as possible after randomization and remained in place for duration of the treating clinician's judgment. The control group was managed without a PAC. Management decisions were at the discretion of the treating clinician. Of note, the participating ICUs could elect to enter one of two strata: not having the option (Stratum A) or having the option (Stratum B) of using alternative cardiac output monitoring in the control group.

Follow-Up: Until hospital discharge.

Endpoints: Primary outcome was in-hospital mortality from any cause. Secondary outcome measures were length of stay in the original ICU, length of stay in the hospital in an acute-ward setting, and organ-days of support required following randomization.

RESULTS

- Hospital mortality was similar in both groups: 66% in the control group and 68% in the PAC group. There was no significant difference in mortality within the ICU and at 28 days between both groups.

- Length of stay in ICU, hospital, and organ-days of support for survivors and non-survivors were similar in both groups
- Complications were noted in 10% (46 of 486) patients of patients in whom PA catheter insertion was attempted. Most commonly these complications were hematomas, arterial puncture, and arrhythmias requiring treatment (Table 12.1).

Table 12.1. SUMMARY OF PAC-MAN KEY FINDINGS

Outcome	PAC N = 506	No PAC N = 507	P Value
Mortality	346 [68%]*	333 [66%]	0.39
ICU Length of Stay, *days*			
Survivors	12.1 [6.2 – 22.3]	11.0 [5.7 – 21.0]	0.26
Non-Survivors	2.6 [0.7 – 8.4]	2.5 [0.8 – 7.2]	0.71

* Numbers are presented as n (%) or median (IQR) depending on type;
PAC: Pulmonary Artery Catheter

Criticisms and Limitations:

- As opposed to the Fluid and Catheter Treatment Trial (FACTT trial, Chapter 23), where the efficacy of PAC use was studied in acute lung injury with rigorous control protocols governing indications for catheterization and management based on data,[2] this was a pragmatic effectiveness trial design where the use of PAC was determined through randomization but very little else was controlled. Thus, it is possible that the negative findings observed in this study resulted from sub-optimal implementation and use of PAC data.
- Patients in this study had a high mortality rate (69%), indicating recruitment of a severely ill population for which management with a PAC may have been unlikely to have had an impact. Thus, the results may not apply to patients that are less ill.
- It has been suggested that the time delay from ICU admission to randomization in the study (median 16 hours) may have been responsible for the lack of benefit. However, a post-hoc secondary analysis revealed no effect on outcome in the quartile of patients randomized within the first 5 hours of ICU admission.

  The majority of ICUs participating (79%) elected to be in Stratum B, which allowed some other form of cardiac output (CO) monitoring device among the control population. In essence, this was a tale of two studies—PAC versus no CO monitor, and PAC versus an alternative CO monitor.

Other Relevant Studies and Information: The PAC has suffered mixed fortunes over the years. The first study that questioned the PAC was a landmark propensity-matched study demonstrating a 24% increased risk of death in patients receiving a PAC within 24 hours of ICU admission.[3] The first randomized controlled trial was published in 2003 demonstrating no mortality or length of stay difference in just under 2000 high-risk older patients undergoing major surgery randomized to goal-directed PAC-guided therapy versus no PAC.[4] Other studies and meta-analyses failed to demonstrate any benefit from PAC use.[5,6] Longitudinal data suggests declining use but significant variability.[7,8]

Summary and Implications: This trial failed to demonstrate a benefit of using PA catheters to manage critically ill patients with respect to mortality or ICU or hospital length of stay. Since PA catheter insertion has risks, the monitor should only be used in select circumstances.

CLINICAL CASE: USE OF THE PULMONARY ARTERY CATHETER

Case History:
A 66-year-old man with a history of coronary artery disease and known ischemic cardiomyopathy is admitted to your ICU following an emergent laparotomy for repair of a ruptured diverticulum. He has a low urine output and continues to require multiple vasopressor medications to maintain a normal blood pressure and perfusion 8 hours postoperatively. Would this patient benefit from insertion of a PA catheter?

Suggested Answer:
The PAC-Man trial demonstrated that there is no clear benefit in managing critically ill patients with a PAC. This patient is similar to the trial patients based in terms of his age, clinical status (multi-organ system disease or decompensated heart failure), and severity of illness. The results of the study suggest that the majority of clinicians using a PAC do so to guide vasoactive or inotropic drug therapy or fluid management without, however, clear benefit in terms of mortality or length of hospital stay. Using noninvasive cardiac output monitoring may be lower risk and provide the same information in this patient.

References

1. Harvey S, Harrison DA, Singer M, et al. Assessment of the clinical effectiveness of pulmonary artery catheters in management of patients in intensive care (PAC-Man): a randomised controlled trial. *Lancet (London, England)*. 2005;366(9484): 472–477.

2. Wheeler AP, Bernard GR, Thompson BT, et al. Pulmonary-artery versus central venous catheter to guide treatment of acute lung injury. *New Engl J Med.* 2006;354(21):2213–2224.
3. Connors AF, Jr., Speroff T, Dawson NV, et al. The effectiveness of right heart catheterization in the initial care of critically ill patients. SUPPORT Investigators. *JAMA.* 1996;276(11):889–897.
4. Sandham JD, Hull RD, Brant RF, et al. A randomized, controlled trial of the use of pulmonary-artery catheters in high-risk surgical patients. *New Engl J Med.* 2003;348(1):5–14.
5. Binanay C, Califf RM, Hasselblad V, et al. Evaluation study of congestive heart failure and pulmonary artery catheterization effectiveness: the ESCAPE trial. *JAMA.* 2005;294(13):1625–1633.
6. Rajaram SS, Desai NK, Kalra A, et al. Pulmonary artery catheters for adult patients in intensive care. *Cochrane Database Syst Rev.* 2013;2:CD003408.
7. Gershengorn HB, Wunsch H. Understanding changes in established practice: pulmonary artery catheter use in critically ill patients. *Crit Care Med.* 2013;41(12):2667–2676.
8. Wiener RS, Welch HG. Trends in the use of the pulmonary artery catheter in the United States, 1993–2004. *JAMA.* 2007;298(4):423–429.

13

Vasopressin versus Norepinephrine Infusion in Patients with Septic Shock

The VASST

KARIM FIKRY

> "Low-dose vasopressin did not reduce mortality rates as compared with norepinephrine among patients with septic shock who were treated with catecholamine vasopressors."
>
> —JA RUSSELL ET AL.

Research Question: Does low-dose vasopressin used as an adjunct to catecholamines decrease mortality among patients with septic shock?[1]

Funding: Supported by a grant from the Canadian Institutes of Health Research.

Year Study Began: 2001

Year Study Published: 2008

Study Location: 27 centers in Canada, Australia, and the United States.

Who Was Studied: Adults (> 16 years of age) who had septic shock that was resistant to fluids and required a minimum of 5 µg of norepinephrine per minute.

Who Was Excluded: Patients with chronic heart disease or unstable coronary syndrome, proven or suspected acute mesenteric ischemia, severe hyponatremia (Na < 130 mmol/L), traumatic brain injury (GCS < 8), pregnancy, malignancy or other irreversible disease where 6-month mortality is >50%, if death was antic-ipated within 12 hours. If open label vasopressin had been used prior to random-ization, patients were excluded. Patients with Raynaud's phenomenon, systemic sclerosis, or vasospastic diathesis were also excluded.

How Many Patients: 6229 patients were screened; 802 patients were random-ized and 778 completed the study.

Study Overview: See Figure 13.1 for an overview of the study design.

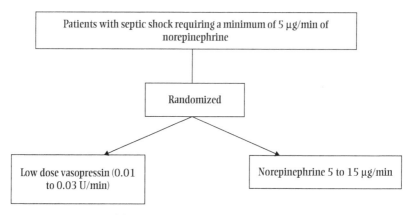

Figure 13.1 Summary of the study design.

Study Intervention: All clinical and research staff, patients, and families were blinded to the study drug. Treatment with either vasopressin or norepinephrine was assigned based on randomization system, which was stratified by center and by severity of shock.

Vasopressin and norepinephrine were mixed in identical 250 mL intravenous bags of 5% dextrose in water, with final concentrations of 0.12 U of vasopressin per milliliter and 60 μg of norepinephrine per milliliter, respectively. The study-drug infusion was started at 5 mL per hour and increased by 2.5 mL per hour every 10 minutes during the first hour to achieve a constant target rate of 15 mL per hour. Titration of the study drug occurred at a constant rate every 10 minutes during the first hour of starting the infusion. The bedside nurse also titrated open-label vaso-pressors to maintain a constant target mean arterial pressure (recommended to be 65 to 75 mm Hg), but it could be modified by the attending ICU physician.

Follow-Up: 90 days

Endpoints: Primary outcome: all-cause mortality at 28 days. Secondary out-comes: 90-day morality; days alive and free of organ dysfunction during the first 28 days; days alive and free of vasopressors, mechanical ventilation, or renal replacement therapy; days alive and free of systemic inflammatory response syndrome; days alive and free of corticosteroid use; length of stay in the ICU and hospital; rates of serious adverse events.

RESULTS

- There were no significant differences in 28-day mortality rate between vasopressin and norepinephrine groups (35.4% and 39.3%, respectively; $p = 0.26$), or 90-day mortality (43.9% and 49.6% respectively; $p = 0.11$)
- Groups did not differ significantly for multiple secondary outcomes including organ dysfunction and length of stay in the ICU and hospital.
- There were no differences in the rates or types of serious adverse events between the two groups.
- In the prospectively defined subgroup of patients with less severe septic shock (requiring 5–14 µg/min of norepinephrine), the mortality rate was lower in the vasopressin group than the norepinephrine group at 28 days (26.5% vs. 35.7%, $p = 0.05$) as well as at 90 days (35.8% vs. 46.1%, $p = 0.04$). However, there was no difference in mortality in the group with more severe septic shock (requiring ≥ 15 µg/min of norepinephrine).

Criticisms and Limitations:

- The study's power calculation was based on an expected mortality of 60%. The lower mortality rate observed in the trial may have resulted in it being underpowered to detect differences between groups. There was a 12 hour randomization delay that may have obscured differences that would have been apparent if the therapies had been initiated immediately.
- Patients were responsive to catecholamines at baseline with mean arterial pressure above 65 mm Hg, making this a study of vasopressin as a "catecholamine-sparing drug" rather than an evaluation in patients who are unresponsive or refractory to catecholamines.
- Only 13% of screened patients were included in the randomization, thus raising the concern that many high-risk patients were excluded, which represents a selection bias. Thus the results may not be generalizable to a "real-world" population.
- Vasopressin levels were not measured which may have served as a guide to the optimal dose or the duration of infusion. A rationale for vasopressin therapy in septic shock is to reduce high, potentially toxic,

catecholamine dosages to ranges with a reasonable benefit–risk ratio. However, the mean norepinephrine dose at randomization in the study was relatively low (0.27 μg per kilogram per minute), and thus little benefit could be expected from lowering catecholamine dosages.

- Patients more likely to benefit from vasopressin-mediated decreases in catecholamine dosages—such as severely sick patients who were expected to die within 12 hours, patients in unstable condition who were receiving vasopressin before study enrollment, and patients with high-risk cardiac disease who were sensitive to catecholamines—were excluded from the trial.

Other Relevant Studies and Information:

- Prior studies have shown that a relative vasopressin deficiency exists in patients with septic shock and therefore administration of vasopressin may be beneficial. Two small randomized trials in patients with septic shock found that vasopressin increased blood pressure, decreased catecholamine requirements, and improved renal function as compared with a control agent. However, neither of the trials was powered to evaluate mortality, organ dysfunction, or safety.
- Post hoc analyses of data from the VASST provide further insights on the results:
- A post hoc substudy of the VASST examined the interaction between vasopressin and corticosteroids and found that the combination was associated with decreased mortality and organ dysfunction compared with norepinephrine and corticosteroids.[2]
- Another post hoc analysis examining cytokine levels from patients enrolled in the VASST found survivors of septic shock had greater decreases of cytokines in early septic shock and that vasopressin decreased 24-hour plasma cytokine levels more than did norepinephrine.[3]
- A post hoc analysis of the cardiopulmonary effects of vasopressin compared with norepinephrine VASST showed that vasopressin treatment was associated with a significant reduction in heart rate but no change in cardiac output or other measures of perfusion.[4]
- A recently published multicenter randomized controlled trial comparing the effect of early use of vasopressin versus norepinephrine on kidney failure in patients with septic shock did not find a difference in kidney failure–free days or mortality.[5]
- A systematic review and meta-analysis of 9 randomized controlled trials evaluating the use of vasopressin and/or terlipressin compared with

catecholamine in adult patients with vasodilatory shock concluded that vasopressin use is safe, associated with reduced mortality, and facilitates weaning of catecholamines.[6] However, a concurrent meta-analysis failed to show a mortality benefit.[7]

- The 2016 Surviving Sepsis Guidelines suggest adding either vasopressin (up to 0.03 U/min) to norepinephrine with the intent of raising mean arterial pressure or adding vasopressin to decrease norepinephrine dosage.[8]

Summary and Implications: This study suggests that in patients with severe septic shock, administration of low-dose vasopressin (up to 0.03 U/min) does not reduce mortality. However, in a subset of patients with less severe septic shock, low-dose vasopressin, in addition to norepinephrine, may have a survival benefit. Since administration of vasopressin was not associated with an increase in adverse events compared to norepinephrine and there is evidence that it may be beneficial in some subgroups of patients, it is reasonable to use it, particularly among patients with catecholamine refractory septic shock.

CLINICAL CASE: ADDITION OF VASOPRESSIN TO NOREPINEPHRINE IN PATIENTS WITH SEPTIC SHOCK

Case History:

A 79-year-old woman with history of COPD is admitted to the ICU with septic shock and ARDS resulting from community acquired pneumonia. She is intubated and mechanically ventilated with tidal volume 400, respiratory rate 24, PEEP 12, and 70% FiO_2. Her blood gas on these ventilator settings is pH 7.21/pCO_2 44/pO_2 59. Despite adequate fluid resuscitation her lactic acid level is 4 mmol/l and her blood pressure is 95/60 on 30 μg/min of norepinephrine. Hydrocortisone is subsequently added for sepsis-related adrenal insufficiency. According to the results of the VASST, would you start concomitant vasopressin infusion on this patient?

Suggested Answer:

Based on the VASST, the addition of vasopressin would not be expected to have a survival benefit for this patient. However, during hypoxic and acidotic conditions the vasoconstrictive effects of vasopressin are better preserved than those of catecholamines such as norepinephrine. Furthermore, post hoc analysis of the trial suggested that in combination with corticosteroids, vasopressin administration was associated with decreased mortality and organ dysfunction. Consequently, it would be appropriate to administer a vasopressin infusion to this patient.

References

1. James A. Russell et al. Vasopressin versus norepinephrine infusion in patients with septic shock. *N Engl J Med*. 2008;358(9):877–887.
2. Russell JA, Walley KR, Gordon AC, et al. Interaction of vasopressin infusion, corticosteroid treatment, and mortality of septic shock. *Crit Care Med*. 2009;37(3):811–818.
3. Russell JA, Fjell C, Hsu JL, et al. Vasopressin compared with norepinephrine augments the decline of plasma cytokine levels in septic shock. *Am J Respir Crit Care Med*. 2013;188:356–364.
4. Gordon AC, Wang N, Walley KR, Ashby D, Russell JA. The cardiopulmonary effects of vasopressin compared with norepinephrine in septic shock. *Chest*. 2012;142(3):593–605.
5. Gordon AC, Mason AJ, Thirunavukkarasu N, et al. Effect of early vasopressin vs norepinephrine on kidney failure in patients with septic shock: the VANISH randomized clinical trial. *JAMA*. 2016;316:509–518.
6. Serpa Neto A, Nassar AP, Cardoso SO, et al. Vasopressin and terlipressin in adult vasodilatory shock: a systematic review and meta-analysis of nine randomized controlled trials. *Crit Care*. 2012;16(4):R154.
7. Polito A, Parisini E, Ricci Z, Picardo S, Annane D. Vasopressin for treatment of vasodilatory shock: an ESICM systematic review and meta-analysis. *Intensive Care Med*. 2012;38(1):9–19.
8. Rhodes A, Evans LE, Alhazzani W, Levy MM, et al. Surviving sepsis campaign: international guidelines for management of sepsis and septic shock: 2016. *Crit Care Med*. 201745(3):486–552.

Comparison of Dopamine and Norepinephrine in the Treatment of Shock

The SOAP II Trial

DANIEL W. JOHNSON

"This study raises serious concerns about the safety of dopamine therapy, since dopamine, as compared with norepinephrine, was associated with more arrhythmias and with an increased rate of death in the subgroup of patients with cardiogenic shock."

—THE SOAP II INVESTIGATORS[1]

Research Question: In the treatment of shock, should dopamine or norepinephrine be the first-line vasopressor agent?[1]

Funding: European Society of Intensive Care through support from the European Critical Care Research Network

Year Study Began: 2003

Year Study Published: 2010

Study Location: 8 centers in Belgium, Austria, and Spain

Who Was Studied: Adults with shock requiring vasopressor therapy. Shock was defined as hypotension (MAP < 70 mm Hg or SBP < 100 mm Hg despite 1000 mL of crystalloid or 500 mL of colloid) in the setting of tissue hypoperfusion (altered mental status, mottled skin, low urine output, or serum lactate ≥ 2 mmol/L).

Who Was Excluded: Patients were excluded if they were under 18 years of age, had already received a vasopressor for more than 4 hours during the current episode of shock, had a serious arrhythmia, or had been declared brain dead.

How Many Patients: 1679

Study Overview: See Figure 14.1 for an overview of the study design.

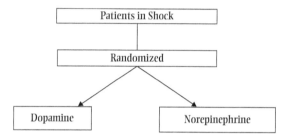

Figure 14.1 Summary of SOAP II design.

Study Intervention: In both groups, target blood pressure was determined by the physician in charge of each patient. Patients in the dopamine group received a weight-based infusion of dopamine that was titrated up and down by 2 mcg/kg/min as needed (maximum of 20 mcg/kg/min). Patients in the norepinephrine group received a weight-based infusion of norepinephrine that was titrated up and down by 0.02 mcg/kg/min as needed (maximum of 0.19 mcg/kg/min).

If the patient remained hypotensive despite maximum dose infusion, open label norepinephrine was added. Epinephrine and vasopressin were used only as rescue therapy. Inotropic agents were used if cardiac output needed to be increased. For weaning, open-label norepinephrine was weaned first, followed by the trial drug. If hypotension recurred, the trial drug was added first, followed by open label norepinephrine.

Follow-Up: 12 months

Endpoints: Primary outcome: mortality rate at 28 days. Secondary outcomes: mortality rates in the ICU and in the hospital, at 6 months and at 12 months.

RESULTS

- There was no significant difference between the dopamine group and the norepinephrine group for any of the key efficacy endpoints (see Table 14.1).

Table 14.1. SUMMARY OF SOAP II's KEY FINDINGS

Outcome	Dopamine group	Norepinephrine group	P value
28-day mortality	52.5%	48.5%	0.10
6-month mortality	63.8%	62.9%	0.71
12-month mortality	65.9%	63.0%	0.34
ICU length of stay	5 days	5 days	0.12
Arrhythmias	24.1%	12.4%	<0.001

- The rate of arrhythmia was significantly higher in the dopamine group (24%) than in the norepinephrine group (12%). Atrial fibrillation accounted for 86% of the arrhythmias.
- Among patients whose shock was cardiogenic in nature, the 28-day mortality was significantly higher in the dopamine group than in the norepinephrine group ($p = 0.03$).
- Among patients whose shock was septic or hypovolemic in nature, there was no significant difference in 28-day mortality between the dopamine group and norepinephrine group.

Criticisms and Limitations:

- Target blood pressure was determined by the physician in charge of treating each patient, so management of this parameter was not standardized. This variability may have confounded the study's findings.
- 26% of patients in the dopamine group and 20% of patients in the norepinephrine group were treated with open-label norepinephrine. These doses (maximum dose of 0.7 and 0.8 µg/kg/min for the dopamine and norepinephrine groups, respectively) were much higher than the maximum dose of norepinephrine (0.16 µg per kilogram per minute) in the norepinephrine group, which might confound the results of the comparison between dopamine and norepinephrine.
- Among patients with septic shock—approximately two thirds of the study population—the early initiation of effective antibiotic therapy and complementary measures for control of the focus of the infection are essential for survival.[2-4] In this study there was no description of whether these measures were implemented similarly in both groups of the protocol.

- Among patients with cardiogenic shock, the study did not describe the proportion of patients in each group that received intraaortic balloon pump support. These data might be relevant to explaining the higher rate of death among patients in cardiogenic shock treated with dopamine, since an intraaortic balloon pump may be helpful in decreasing the need for inotropic support, thus reducing the potential risk of arrhythmias.

Other Relevant Studies and Information:

- In a large population-based sample of patients with septic shock in the United States, use of norepinephrine as initial vasopressor was associated with a small but significant mortality benefit over dopamine.[3]
- A 2016 Cochrane Review of 28 studies that compared individual vasopressors to other vasopressors concluded that dopamine increases risk of arrhythmias and might increase risk of mortality compared with norepinephrine. Evidence was insufficient to define other differences between vasopressors.[4]
- The Surviving Sepsis Campaign's 2016 update recommends norepinephrine as the first-line vasopressor in the treatment of septic shock. Dopamine is suggested as an alternative vasopressor agent to norepinephrine only in highly selected patients (e.g., patients with low risk of tachyarrhythmia and absolute or relative bradycardia).[5]

Summary and Implications: This large randomized trial did not identify a mortality difference between dopamine and norepinephrine for patients in shock, but the rate of arrhythmia was significantly higher in the dopamine group than in the norepinephrine group. Among patients whose shock was cardiogenic in nature, the 28-day mortality was significantly higher in the dopamine group than in the norepinephrine group. This and other studies prompted the Surviving Sepsis Campaign to recommend norepinephrine as the first-line vasopressor for septic shock and the American College of Cardiology and the American Heart Association to stop recommending dopamine as a first-line agent for post-STEMI cardiogenic shock.[6,7]

CLINICAL CASE: DOPAMINE VERSUS NOREPINEPHRINE AS FIRST-LINE VASOPRESSOR FOR SHOCK

Case History:
A 68-year-old man with hypertension and mild chronic obstructive pulmonary disease (COPD) presents to the emergency department with lethargy and bladder pain. Vital signs include temperature = 38.9°C,

heart rate = 93, respiratory rate = 30, blood pressure = 72/34 mm Hg and SpO_2 = 91% on air. The white blood cell count is 18,000 and an ECG reveals sinus rhythm with frequent premature atrial complexes (PACs). Despite fluid resuscitation and administration of antibiotics, the patient remains hypotensive with low urine output. Based on the results of this study, how should this patient be treated?

Suggested Answer:

This study showed that for patients in shock, there was an increased risk of arrhythmias with dopamine administration compared with norepinephrine. This patient presents with classic septic shock secondary to urinary tract infection. The elevated heart rate, frequent PACs, and history of hypertension and COPD suggest an increased risk for arrhythmia. Because of these risk factors for arrhythmia, norepinephrine—not dopamine—would be the preferred agent to maintain the blood pressure.

References

1. De Backer D, Biston P, Devriendt J, et al. for the SOAP II Investigators. Comparison of dopamine and norepinephrine in the treatment of shock. *N Engl J Med.* 2010;362:779–789.

2. Dellinger RP, Carlet JM, Masur H, et al. for the Surviving Sepsis Campaign Management Guidelines Committee. Surviving Sepsis Campaign guidelines for management of severe sepsis and septic shock. *Crit Care Med.* 2004;32(3):858–873.

3. Fawzy A, Evans SR, Walkey AJ. Practice patterns and outcomes associated with choice of initial vasopressor therapy for septic shock. *Crit Care Med.* 2015;43(10):2141–2146.

4. Gamper G, Havel C, Arrich J, Losert H, Pace NL, Mullner M, Herkner H. Vasopressors for hypotensive shock. *Cochrane Database Syst Rev.* 2016;Issue 2. Art. No.:CD003709.

5. Rhodes A, Evans LE, Alhazzani W et al. Surviving Sepsis Campaign: international guidelines for management of sepsis and septic shock: 2016.*Crit Care Med.* 2017;45(3):486–552.

6. Antman EM, Anbe DT, Armstrong PW et al. for the ACC/AHA Writing Committee Members. ACC/AHA Guidelines for the management of patients with ST-elevation myocardial infarction—executive summary. *Circulation.* 2004;110(5):588–636.

7. O'Gara PT, Kushner FG, Ascheim DD, et al. for the ACCF/AHA task force on practice guidelines. 2013 ACCF/AHA *Guideline for* the management of ST-elevation myocardial infarction. *J Am Coll Cardiol.* 2013;61(4):e78–140.

15

CPR with Chest Compression Alone or with Rescue Breathing

CHRISTOPHER "KIT" TAINTER AND GABRIEL WARDI

"[A strategy of compression-only CPR in out-of-hospital cardiac arrest] ... viewed within the context of other investigations, strengthen[s] a layperson CPR strategy that emphasizes chest compression and minimizes the role of rescue breathing."

—THOMAS REA ET AL.

Research Question: In patients with out-of-hospital cardiac arrest receiving bystander cardiopulmonary resuscitation (CPR), does a compression-only strategy lead to improved survival to hospital discharge when compared to the traditional compression and rescue breath strategy?[1]

Funding: The Laerdal Foundation for Acute Medicine and the Medic One Foundation.

Year Study Began: 2005

Year Study Published: 2010

Study Locations: Two counties in Washington State, United States, and London, England.

Who Was Studied: Patients were eligible if the dispatcher determined that they were unconscious and not breathing normally, bystander CPR was not already under way, and if the caller was willing to undertake CPR with the dispatcher's assistance.

Who Was Excluded: Patients who were unconscious and not breathing normally but who were determined not to be in cardiac arrest, persons who had had a confirmed arrest but had signs of irreversible death, in which case EMS personnel did not attempt resuscitation. In addition, patients with arrest due to trauma, drowning, or asphyxiation, as well as patients who were under 18 years of age; and those who had do-not-resuscitate status or were already receiving CPR were also excluded.

How Many Patients: 1941

Study Overview: See Figure 15.1 for an overview of the study design.

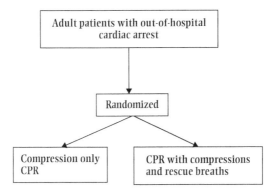

Figure 15.1 Summary of the study design.

Study Intervention: On determining patients' eligibility, the bystander was then randomly assigned to a study group and instructed to perform either chest compressions alone (50 consecutive compressions, one cycle), or chest compressions plus rescue breathing, with 2 initial rescue breaths followed by 15 chest compressions and subsequent cycles continuing the pattern in a ratio of 2 to 15. For the two sites in the United States, resuscitation was guided by the American Heart Association (AHA) guidelines whereas the site in the United Kingdom followed the United Kingdom Resuscitation Council (UKRC) guidelines.

Follow-Up: Enrolled subjects were followed from time of EMS activation until either they were discharged from the hospital or died.

Endpoints: The primary outcome in this trial was survival to hospital discharge. Secondary endpoints included return of spontaneous circulation at the end of EMS care and favorable neurologic status at the time of hospital discharge, defined as a Cerebral Performance Category (CPC) of 1 or 2.

RESULTS

- 12.5% of patients survived in the compression-only group versus 11.0% in the compression and rescue breath group ($p = 0.31$).
- Arrests from a cardiac cause had improved neurologic outcomes in the compression-only group (18.9% versus 13.5%, $p = 0.03$).
- A shockable rhythm was associated with a trend toward survival to hospital discharge in the compression-only group (31.9% versus 25.7%, $p = 0.09$).
- For those with a non-cardiac cause of arrest, there was no difference in survival between the compression-only and traditional CPR groups (5.0% versus 7.2%, $p = 0.29$) (Table 15.1).

Table 15.1. SUMMARY OF STUDY'S KEY FINDINGS

Outcome	Compressions only CPR	Compressions and rescue breath CPR	p value
Survival to Hospital discharge	12.5%	11.0%	0.31
Favorable neurologic status	14.4%	11.5%	0.13
Survival with underlying cardiac cause of arrest	15.5%	12.3%	0.09

Criticisms and Limitations:

- Although the study enrolled almost 2000 patients, it may still have had insufficient power to detect clinically important differences. For example, the study would need approximately 4200 subjects to have 80% power to demonstrate a significant difference in survival with a favorable neurologic outcome between the 2 study groups (assuming 14.4% for chest compression alone and 11.5% for chest compression plus rescue breathing).
- Certain common causes of cardiac arrest were excluded (e.g., patients who arrested from asphyxiation, drowning, and trauma), which may limit the generalizability of the results.
- CPR in the rescue breath group was performed with a compression to rescue breath ratio of 15:2. This ratio that is no longer recommended by the American Heart Association, which now recommends a strategy of 30 compressions for every 2 rescue breaths.[2]
- The study investigated CPR performed by bystanders. The results may not apply to health professionals, who are more practiced and proficient in CPR, often engaging at a later stage of arrest physiology. Also, the results may not necessarily apply to trained bystanders.

Other Relevant Studies and Information: Out-of-hospital cardiac arrest is a major public health concern in the United States, with around 300,000 episodes per year in the United States with less than 10% surviving to hospital discharge.[3] The physiologic benefit of compression-only CPR has been shown in numerous animal studies and likely results from both improved coronary perfusion pressure and increased venous return. Both interruptions of chest compressions during ventilation and positive-pressure ventilations have been demonstrated to have detrimental effects on survival rate. Furthermore, many bystanders have reservations about performing mouth-to-mouth rescue breathing and are therefore deterred from initiating CPR. In addition, compression-only CPR is easier to teach, remember, and perform, qualities that may result in more bystanders willing to perform CPR and more effective chest compressions.

- A systematic review and meta-analysis was performed by Hüpfl et al. that compared compression-only CPR with the traditional compression and rescue breath.[4] Pooling of three randomized controlled trials (RCTs) with compression-only CPR conducted by a dispatcher-assisted bystander demonstrated an absolute survival increase of 2.4% (NNT 41) versus standard CPR with compressions and rescue breaths. These RCTs preferentially included arrests from a cardiac cause, thus making the findings difficult to generalize to other causes. When the analysis was expanded to include all causes of cardiac arrest with 7 additional observational trials, no difference was seen between compression-only CPR and standard CPR.
- A recently published 5-year prospective statewide observational study in Arizona showed that training the population in continuous chest compressions until the arrival of emergency medical services (EMS) increased the rate of bystander-initiated CPR and increased the rate of survival to discharge from the hospital.[5]
- A recent randomized trial of 23,711 adult patients with non–trauma-related cardiac arrest treated by EMS providers compared continuous chest compressions with chest compressions interrupted by rescue breathing.[6] The study did not find significantly higher rates of survival or favorable neurologic function in the compression-only group compared with the interrupted chest compressions, a finding that may reflect that the deleterious effects of rescue breathing are diminished when "high-quality" CPR is administered by experienced providers.

Summary and Implications: This study suggest that for patients with out-of-hospital cardiac arrest due to cardiac causes and receiving bystander CPR, there is no added benefit to rescue breaths interposed with chest compressions if EMS arrives quickly. The 2015 American Heart Association guidelines now recommend compression-only CPR for untrained bystanders, although rescue breaths are still recommended for those who have undergone prior training at a ratio of 30 compressions to 2 rescue breaths.[2]

CLINICAL CASE: COMPRESSION-ONLY CPR FOR OUT-OF-HOSPITAL CARDIAC ARREST

Case History:
A 55-year-old male grasps his chest and suddenly falls to the ground at a family gathering. It is found that he has no pulse, and 9-1-1 is immediately called. No one present has undergone CPR training. What approach to CPR should be recommended for this patient?

Suggested Answer:
This study, as well as several others, suggest for untrained bystanders a compression-only approach to CPR is appropriate. It is likely that this man's arrest had a cardiac cause, and the compression-only approach may provide additional benefit for both his chances of survival and a favorable neurological outcome. Furthermore, bystanders are more likely to initiate a compression-only approach, especially if untrained in CPR.

References

1. Rea TD, Fahrenbruch C, Culley L, et al. "CPR with chest compression alone or with rescue breathing." *New Engl J Med.* 2010;363(5):423–433.
2. Neumar RW, Shuster M, Callaway CW. Part 1: Executive summary: 2015 American Heart Association Guidelines update for cardiopulmonary resuscitation and emergency cardiovascular care. *Circulation.* 2015;132:S315–S367.
3. Lloyd-Jones D, Adams R, Carnethon M, et al., American Heart Association Statistics Committee and Stroke Statistics Subcommittee. Heart disease and stroke statistics, 2009 update: a report from the American Heart Association Statistics Committee and Stroke Statistics Subcommittee. *Circulation.* 2009;119(3):480–486.
4. Hüpfl M, Selig HF, Nagele P. Chest-compression-only versus standard cardiopulmonary resuscitation: a meta-analysis. *Lancet.* 2010;376(9752):1552–1557.
5. Bobrow BJ, Spaite DW, Berg RA. Chest compression-only CPR by lay rescuers and survival from out-of-hospital cardiac arrest. *JAMA.* 2010;304(13):1447–1454.
6. Nichol G, Leroux B, Wang H. Trial of continuous or interrupted chest compressions during CPR. *N Engl J Med.* 2015;373:2203–2214.

Advanced Heart Failure Treated with Continuous-Flow Left Ventricular Assist Device

DAVID M. DUDZINSKI AND JAMES SAWALLA GUSEH

"[C]ontinuous-flow, permanent left ventricular assist device therapy in selected patients as a means to provide long term hemodynamic support […] is linked to improvements in longevity and the quality of life."

—SLAUGHTER ET AL.

Research Question: How does a second-generation *continuous*-flow left ventricular assist device compare with a first generation *pulsatile*-flow device with regard to the clinical endpoints of survival, freedom from stroke, and freedom from device exchange?[1]

Funding: Thoratec Corporation

Year Study Began: 2005

Year Study Published: 2009

Study Location: 38 centers in the United States

Who Was Studied: Medically refractory patients with advanced heart failure, defined as having a "left ventricular ejection fraction less than 25%; a peak VO_2 consumption of less than 14 mL/kg or less than 50% predicted, NYHA Class IIIB or IV, 7 days of intra-aortic balloon pump dependence, or 14 days of inotrope dependence."[1] The vast majority of patients (> 75%) were receiving concomitant intravenous inotropes.

Who Was Excluded: Excluded patients were those thought to have irreversible organ failure defined as "severe renal, pulmonary, or hepatic dysfunction," or active infection.

How Many Patients: 200 patients were randomized to continuous-flow and pulsatile-flow left ventricular assist devices (LVADs) at a 2:1 ratio (See Figure 16.1). Ultimately 134 patients received a continuous flow LVAD while 66 patients received a pulsatile flow device.

Study Overview: Patients were screened before randomization for severe and medically refractory advanced heart failure, and enrolled patients were randomized to receive one of two types of left ventricular assist devices: either the pulsatile HeartMate XVE device versus a continuous flow HeartMate II device, both created by Thoratec Corporation.

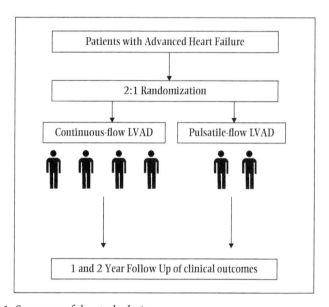

Figure 16.1 Summary of the study design.

The overall analysis was centered on a primary composite endpoint of survival, freedom from disabling stroke and freedom from repeat operation. Many other clinically relevant end points were also followed in the two populations.

Study Intervention: The dominant and existing left ventricular assist device prior to this clinical trial was the HeartMate XVE which was a 450 mL, 1250-gram device with a pulsatile flow mechanism, where blood was ejected in boluses out of the device by a pumping displacement mechanism. Patients randomized to this device were receiving standard of care. These patients, importantly, were not anticoagulated.

The study intervention was randomization to a second-generation left ventricular assist device known as the HeartMate II which had significantly less volume (63 mL) and mass (390 grams). In contrast to the first-generation HeartMate XVE, the HeartMate II had a continuous flow mechanism. This continuous flow device is a high-speed rotary pump that delivers axial flow, and has the promise of improved hemodynamics and end-organ function, as well as enhanced mechanical durability making them more useful for long-term patient support. Patients receiving continuous flow LVAD underwent systemic anticoagulation with warfarin for an international normalized ratio goal of 2.0 to 3.0.

Both devices had the capacity to generate 10 liters/minute of flow with a mean pressure of 100 mm Hg. Background therapy included aspirin for all patients.

Follow-Up: 2 years

Endpoints: Primary endpoint: A composite of two-year survival, freedom from disabling stroke characterized by a Rankin score >3, and freedom from reoperation to replace the device. Secondary endpoints included actuarial survival, adverse event frequency, quality of life metrics, and functional status.

RESULTS

Primary Endpoints Achieved:
Patients with the continuous flow LVAD achieved improved outcomes vs. those with pulsatile flow LVAD (primary endpoint 46% vs. 11%, respectively, $p < 0.001$, see Table 16.1). The difference was driven predominantly by a reduced need for reoperation, replacement, or repair of the device.

Table 16.1. PRINCIPAL FINDINGS ACCORDING TO TREATMENT ARM

Outcome	Continuous Flow LVAD N = 134	Pulsatile Flow LVAD N = 66	P Value
2 Year actuarial survival	58%	24%	0.008
Composite endpoint of freedom from death, stroke, and need for reoperation or repair at 2 years	46% ($n = 62$ of 134)	11% ($n = 7$ of 66)	< 0.001
First composite event			
Death, within 2 years of LVAD implantation	33%	41%	0.048
Disabling stroke	11%	12%	0.56
Repair/reoperation to replace LVAD	10%	36%	< 0.001

Hemodynamic Improvements:
- 2.0 to 2.9 L/minute/m^2 improvement in cardiac index (continuous flow)
- 2.1 to 2.9 L/minute//m^2 improvement in cardiac index (pulsatile flow)
- Pulmonary capillary wedge pressure decreased from 24 mm Hg to 17 mm Hg (pulsatile flow) and 24 mm Hg to 16 mm Hg (continuous flow)

Actuarial Survival:
- The one year Kaplan-Meier survival curve estimates were 68% for continuous flow devices and 55% for the pulsatile-flow device.
- The two-year Kaplan-Meier survival curve estimate was 58% for the continuous flow device and 24% for the pulsatile-flow device.

Functional Status:
There were significant improvements in functional status enjoyed by both groups.

- 80% of patients with a continuous-flow LVAD had NYHA functional class I or II symptoms at 24 months.
- There were significant improvements in 6-minute walk distances in both study groups suggesting that the exercise benefits are related to the reduction of cardiac filling pressures and improvement in cardiac output rather than being related to the characteristics of either pulsatile or continuous flow.
- Validated questionnaires also indicated significant improvements in quality of life in both groups.
- There was a 38% relative reduction in the rate of rehospitalization among patients with a continuous-flow LVAD as compared with those with a pulsatile-flow device. Total time outside the hospital after LVAD insertion was 88% for the continuous device versus 74% with the pulsatile LVAD ($p = 0.02$).

Adverse Events:
The continuous flow pump fared better than the pulsatile flow pump with regard to the adverse events profile. There were reduced rates of pump replacement as well as fewer thrombotic and infectious complications. There was less right heart failure as well as decreased rates of organ failure enjoyed by patients on the continuous flow pumps. The patients with a continuous flow pump also had lower rates of rehospitalization.

Criticisms and Limitations: The trial was non-blinded and patients could appreciate the difference simply by the noise and weight of the implanted device, potentially biasing patient-reported outcomes. Additionally, the authors did not report how much pre-screening was conducted to achieve sufficient numbers for randomization. Additionally, trial patients were specifically selected that had a low-to-medium risk mean destination therapy risk score (predictive of a probability of survival to hospital discharge of more than 70%). Therefore, it is unclear as to whether the results can be applied to the general population of patients with heart failure.

Other Relevant Studies and Information:

- This study expanded the literature and experience of mechanical support devices and added to the seminal REMATCH Trial[2] which was the first large study to demonstrate a role for mechanical support in patients with advanced heart failure not eligible for transplant. Pulsatile LVADs, when compared with medical therapy, showed a 48% mortality reduction. One year survival was boosted from 25 to 52% with a device and two-year survival boosted from 8 to 23%. The FDA approved LVAD therapy based upon these findings.[3]
- The HeartMate II continuous flow device had previously been shown to be effective hemodynamic support for patients awaiting heart transplantation however until the Slaughter trial had never been directly compared with pulsatile LVAD technology.[4]
- As there has been increasing usage of these LVADs, The Interagency Registry for Mechanically Assisted Circulatory Support (InterMACS) was created to collect clinical data on mechanically assisted patients. The optimal candidates for LVAD support have been refined based upon clinical data generated from this registry and others.[5,6]
- The ROADMAP study[7] was a 200-patient prospective observational multicenter trial comparing the use of a continuous flow LVAD against medical therapy in ambulatory patients. It was unique because it examined ambulatory inotrope-independent advanced heart failure patients. It demonstrated a 1-year mortality benefit (80 v. 63%; $p = 0.024$) and an improvement in the quality of life in advanced heart failure outpatients undergoing LVAD placement.
- Continuous-flow left ventricular assist devices (LVAD) have emerged as the standard of care for advanced heart failure patients requiring long-term mechanical circulatory support.[8] The field continues to innovate around LVAD design and technology aspiring to engineer safer, more durable pumps for patients with advanced heart failure.[9]

Summary and Implications: In patients with advanced systolic heart failure, the use of a continuous-flow LVAD dramatically improved the likelihood of survival (actuarial two year survival, and event-free survival) when compared to a pulsatile-flow LVAD—particularly for those patients who are inotrope dependent. LVADs reduce mortality while improving functional status, time out of the hospital, and quality of life. Continuous flow LVADs also required ~1/8 the need for pump replacements compared to the pulsatile flow LVADs. LVADs, however, are not without risk including cerebral thromboembolism, and are only appropriate in carefully selected patients with advanced heart failure requiring advanced therapy, such as continuous inotropic support.

CLINICAL CASE: REFRACTORY HEART FAILURE DESPITE CARDIAC RESYNCHRONIZATION THERAPY AND CONTINUOUS INOTROPIC THERAPY

Case History:

A 62-year-old man with ischemic cardiomyopathy and left ventricle ejection fraction 15% is admitted with advanced acute on chronic systolic heart failure (NYHA Class IIIB symptomatology) that has progressed inexorably for the last 4 months despite cardiac resynchronization therapy and home inotropes. His blood pressure is 100/60 mm Hg and he cannot tolerate ACE inhibitor therapy due to hypotension. He is deemed ineligible for cardiac transplantation. He had undergone CRT 6 months prior but has neither experienced clinical benefit nor reverse remodeling by echocardiography. His 6-minute walk distance is 180 meters and he is dependent on dobutamine and milrinone. Based on the results of the study, what specific therapy might be offered?

Suggested Answer:

Continuous inotropic support helps patients with advanced heart failure in the short term but the 1 year survival rate is less than 10–30%. Prior investigations suggested that patients with advanced heart failure and certain clinical characteristics have improved outcomes with pulsatile-flow left ventricular assist devices as compared with medical therapy. Based on the study by Slaughter, this patient would benefit from evaluation for mechanical circulatory support; in the Slaughter patient population CRT had previously failed in more than 60%, and continuous inotropes were being used in 80% of patients. If amenable, specific recommendations would be for a continuous-flow LVAD, which proved more effective than a pulsatile device in this study. A continuous device was associated with a mortality benefit, an improved adverse events profile, improved functional status and an improved quality of life versus pulsatile-flow LVAD. These benefits would have to be balanced with risks of post-LVAD bleeding, stroke, infection, and repeat procedures.

References

1. Slaughter MS, Rogers JG, Milano CA, et al. Advanced heart failure treated with continuous-flow left ventricular assist device. *N Engl J Med*. 2009;361(23):2241–2251. doi:10.1056/NEJMoa0909938.

2. Rose EA, Gelijns AC, Moskowitz AJ, et al. Long-term use of a left ventricular assist device for end-stage heart failure. *N Engl J Med*. 2001;345(20):1435–1443. doi:10.1056/NEJMoa012175.

3. Fang JC. Rise of the machines: left ventricular assist devices as permanent therapy for advanced heart failure. *N Engl J Med*. 2009;361(23):2282–2285. doi:10.1056/NEJMe0910394.

4. Miller LW, Pagani FD, Russell SD, et al. Use of a continuous-flow device in patients awaiting heart transplantation. *N Engl J Med*. 2007;357(9):885–896. doi:10.1056/NEJMoa067758.

5. Stevenson LW, Pagani FD, Young JB, et al. INTERMACS profiles of advanced heart failure: the current picture. *J Heart Lung Transplant*. 2009;28(6):535–541. doi:10.1016/j.healun.2009.02.015.

6. Holman WL, Kormos RL, Naftel DC, et al. Predictors of death and transplant in patients with a mechanical circulatory support device: a multi-institutional study. *J Heart Lung Transplant*. 2009;28(1):44–50. doi:10.1016/j.healun.2008.10.011.

7. Estep JD, Starling RC, Horstmanshof DA, et al. Risk assessment and comparative effectiveness of left ventricular assist device and medical management in ambulatory heart failure patients results from the ROADMAP study. *J Am Coll Cardiol*. 2015;66(16):1747–1761. doi:10.1016/j.jacc.2015.07.075.

8. Slaughter MS, Pagani FD, Rogers JG, et al. Clinical management of continuous-flow left ventricular assist devices in advanced heart failure. *J Heart Lung Transplant*. 2010;29(4 Suppl):S1–39.

9. Mehra MR, Naka Y, Uriel N, et al. A Fully Magnetically Levitate Circulatory Pump for Advanced Heart Failure. *N Engl J Med*. 2017:376: 440–450. doi: 10.1056/NEJMoa1610426.

17

Intraaortic Balloon Support in Myocardial Infarction Complicated by Cardiogenic Shock

SAMUEL BERNARD AND DAVID M. DUDZINSKI

" . . . in patients with cardiogenic shock complicating myocardial infarction for whom early revascularization was planned . . . use of intraaortic balloon pump counterpulsation, as compared with conventional therapy, did not reduce 30-day mortality."

—THIELE ET AL.

Research Question: Compared to optimal medical therapy (OMT) alone, does intraaortic balloon pump (IABP) counterpulsation reduce mortality in patients with acute myocardial infarction (MI) complicated by cardiogenic shock in whom early revascularization in planned?[1]

Sponsors: German Research Foundation and unrestricted grants from Maquet Cardiopulmonary and Teleflex Medical

Year Study Began: 2009

Year Study Published: 2012

Study Location: 37 centers in Germany

Who Was Studied: Patients 18–90 years old presenting with cardiogenic shock complicating acute MI (with or without ST-segment elevation) with planned revascularization (either percutaneous coronary intervention [PCI] or coronary artery bypass grafting [CABG]). Patients were considered to be in cardiogenic shock if they had a systolic blood pressure (SBP) < 90 mm Hg for 30 minutes or needed catecholamine infusion to maintain SBP, had signs of pulmonary congestion, and had signs of end organ hypoperfusion.

Who Was Excluded: Exclusion criteria for this trial included age > 90 years, shock of a non-cardiogenic etiology (sepsis, pulmonary embolism), shock duration > 12 hours before screening, patients with prolonged periods of resuscitation (> 30 minutes), asystole, profound cerebral deficits after resuscitation, severe peripheral arterial disease, greater than grade II aortic regurgitation (on a scale of I to IV), or life expectancy < 6 months.

How Many Patients: 600

Study Overview: See Figure 17.1 for an overview of the study design.

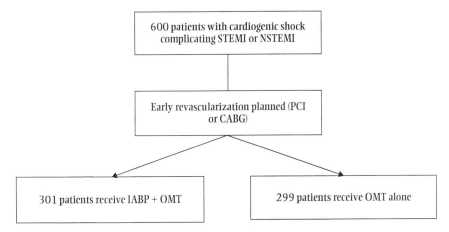

Figure 17.1 Summary of the IABP-SHOCK II design.

Study Intervention: Patients were randomized to IABP counterpulsation with OMT versus OMT alone.[2] IABP was inserted before or immediately after revascularization. 1:1 electrocardiographic IABP triggering was maintained until there was hemodynamic stability (defined as a SBP >90 mm Hg for 30 minutes without the need of vasopressor medications). Patient crossover was allowed only if there was interval development of a mechanical complication of MI—ventricular septal defect or papillary muscle rupture.

Patients underwent revascularization by primary PCI of the target lesion, PCI of the target lesion with additional immediate or staged PCI of nontarget lesions, or CABG, at the discretion of the interventionalist. Remaining ICU care was at the discretion of the intensivist.

Follow-Up: 30 days

Endpoints: The primary study endpoint was 30-day all-cause mortality. Safety end points included in-hospital bleeding (severe, life-threatening, or moderate), peripheral ischemic complications requiring surgical or interventional therapy, sepsis, and stroke.

RESULTS

- 10% of patients randomized to the control arm received an IABP and 4.3% of patients randomized to IABP + OMT did not receive the device.
- There were no differences in 30-day mortality between groups in the intention-to-treat, per-protocol or as-treated analyses (Table 17.1).
- These results were consistent across all prespecified subgroups including patients with STEMI versus NSTEMI and those who received IABP before or after revascularization.
- There were also no significant differences in safety end points between the two groups (Table 17.1).

Table 17.1. PRIMARY AND SAFETY OUTCOMES OF THE IABP-SHOCK II TRIAL

Outcome	IABP (n = 300)	Control (n = 298)	P-Value
All-cause mortality (30 days, primary end point)	39.7%	41.3%	0.69
Stroke	0.7%	1.7%	0.28
Ischemic	0.7%	1.3%	0.45
Hemorrhagic	0%	0.3%	0.50
Peripheral ischemic complications requiring intervention in hospital	4.3%	3.4%	0.53
Bleeding, in hospital			
Life threatening or severe	3.3%	4.4%	0.51
Moderate	17.3%	16.4%	0.77
Sepsis in hospital	15.7%	20.5%	0.15

Criticisms and Limitations:

- The trial was powered based on an estimated 44% mortality rate in the control group. Given the lower observed mortality, it was suggested that the study was underpowered.[3]
- Roughly 90% of patients were on catecholamines when enrolled and 50% had an SBP of >90 mm Hg. Use of catecholamines themselves

could worsen myocardial dysfunction through increased afterload and myocardial ischemia, thereby diminishing efficacy of IABP.[4,5]

- 25% of patients presented with a right coronary artery (RCA) infarction, which could have generated right ventricular dysfunction and potential confounding for the utility of IABP placement.[6]
- 10% of patients in the control group received IABP therapy in violation of the protocol. This cross-over may have affected the study results. However, the per-protocol analysis (which analyzes patients according to the treatment they received rather than the treatment they were assigned to) failed to demonstrate a benefit with IABP. Furthermore, the as-treated analysis also did not show a benefit.

Other Relevant Studies and Information:

- At 12-month follow-up, there remained no differences in all-cause mortality, reinfarction, repeat revascularization, or stroke.[7]
- In post-hoc analyses of IABP-SHOCK II, IABP placement was associated with higher health care costs, but no statistically significant differences in quality of life or functional class at 12 months of follow-up.[8] Moreover, there were no differences in mortality of men versus women at 1 day, 30 days, 6 months, and 12 months of follow-up when multivariable adjustment was performed.[9]
- A meta-analysis of patients with acute MI complicated by cardiogenic shock suggests that IABP may have a beneficial effect on some hemodynamic parameters, but there was no survival benefit.[10]
- A 2015 SCAI/ACC/HFSA/STS Clinical Expert Consensus Statement on the Use of Percutaneous Mechanical Circulatory Support Devices concluded that "In the setting of profound cardiogenic shock, IABP is less likely to provide benefit than continuous flow pumps including the Impella CP and TandemHeart."[11]

Summary and Implications: In patients with acute MI complicated by cardiogenic shock who are undergoing early revascularization, the addition of IABP to OMT results in no mortality benefit. These findings suggest IABP may not have a role in treatment of this patient population. However, IABP placement did not appear to worsen safety outcomes, and in practice it is still considered among the mechanical circulatory support options for salvage or rescue.

CLINICAL CASE: INTRAAORTIC BALLOON PUMP IN THE TREATMENT OF MYOCARDIAL INFARCTION AND CARDIOGENIC SHOCK

Case History:

A 68-year-old man with diabetes, hypertension, and a 100-pack-year smoking history presents to the emergency room with 15 minutes of crushing substernal chest pain, diaphoresis, and shortness of breath. Initial vital signs are BP 80/50, HR 103, O_2 saturation 86% on ambient air. Electrocardiogram shows 3 mm ST-elevations in leads V1–V4. The patient is taken urgently to cardiac catheterization wherein an occlusive thrombus of the proximal LAD is identified. After stent placement, the patient's blood pressure is 72/46. You are asked if an intraaortic balloon pump should be placed while the patient is in the angiography suite. Based on the results of the IABP-SHOCK II trial, how should you proceed?

Suggested Answer:

This study suggests that insertion of an IABP would provide no mortality benefit for this patient at 30 days (and at 12 months based on follow-up studies). However, there is some suggestion from meta-analyses that hemodynamics are improved in the short-term with IABP placement. Ultimately this requires result judgment by the intensivist—if the patient's hemodynamics are rapidly deteriorating before further medical therapy can be provided, IABP may be reasonable to consider for left ventricle unloading or other short-term clinical goals.

References

1. Thiele H, Zeymer U, Neumann FJ, et al. Intraaortic balloon support for myocardial infarction with cardiogenic shock. *N Engl J Med.* 2012;367(14):1287–1296.
2. Thiele H, Schuler G, Neumann F-J, et al. Intraaortic balloon counterpulsation in acute myocardial infarction complicated by cardiogenic shock: design and rationale of the Intraaortic Balloon Pump in Cardiogenic Shock II (IABP-SHOCK II) trial. *Am Heart J.* 2012;163:938–945.
3. Perera D, Lumley M, Pijls N, et al. Intra-aortic balloon trials: Questions, answered, and unresolved issues. *Circulation: Cardio Intervent.* 2013;6:317–321.
4. Kleber FX. Intraaortic balloon support for cardiogenic shock. *N Engl J Med.* 2013;368(1):80.
5. Rekhraj S, Noman A. Intraaortic balloon support for cardiogenic shock. *N Engl J Med.* 2013;368(1):80–81.
6. Kleber FX. Intraaortic balloon support for cardiogenic shock. *N Engl J Med.* 2013;368(1):80.

7. Thiele H, Zeymer U, Neumann FJ, et al. Intra-aortic balloon counterpulsation in acute myocardial infarction complicated by cardiogenic shock (IABP-SHOCK II): final 12 month results of a randomised, open-label trial. *Lancet.* 2013;382(9905): 1638–1645.
8. Schuster A, Faulkner M, Zeymer U, et al. Economic implications of intra-aortic balloon support for myocardial infarction with cardiogenic shock: an analysis from the IABP-SHOCK II-trial. *Clin Res Cardiol.* 2015;104(7):566–573.
9. Fengler K, Fuernau G, Desch S, et al. Gender differences in patients with cardiogenic shock complicating myocardial infarction: a substudy of the IABP-SHOCK II-trial. *Clin Res Cardiol.* 2015;104(1):71–78.
10. Unverzagt S, Buerke M, de Waha A, et al. Intra-aortic balloon pump counterpulsation (IABP) for myocardial infarction complicated by cardiogenic shock. *Cochrane Database Syst Rev.* 2015;3:CD007398.
11. Rihal CS, Naidu SS, Givertz MM, et al. 2015 SCAI/ACC/HFSA/STS clinical expert consensus statement on the use of percutaneous mechanical circulatory support devices in cardiovascular care: Endorsed by the American Heart Association, the Cardiological Society of India, and Sociedad Latino Americana de Cardiologia Intervencion; Affirmation of Value by the Canadian Association of Interventional Cardiology-Association Canadienne de Cardiologie d'intervention. *J Am Coll Cardiol.* 2015;65(19):e7–e26.

18

Angioplasty versus Fibrinolytics in Acute ST-Elevation Myocardial Infarction

The DANAMI-2 Trial

BRYAN SIMMONS

> " . . . primary angioplasty is superior to fibrinolysis for patients who have myocardial infarction with ST-segment elevation, even when patients are admitted to a local hospital . . . and must be transported to an invasive-treatment center,"
> —THE DANAMI-2 INVESTIGATORS

Research Question: In hospitals without angioplasty capabilities, should patients presenting with acute ST-elevation myocardial infarction (STEMI) be managed with onsite fibrinolysis or transferred to the nearest facility for primary angioplasty?[1]

Sponsor: Danish Heart Foundation, Danish Medical Research Council, AstraZeneca, Bristol-Myers Squibb, Cordis, Pfizer, Pharmacia-Upjohn, Boehringer Ingelheim, and Guerbet.

Year Study Began: 1997

Year Study Published: 2003

Study Location: 29 hospitals in Denmark—24 referral hospitals without angioplasty facilities and 5 hospitals with angioplasty capabilities.

Who Was Studied: Patients at least 18 years of age presenting with symptoms consistent with myocardial infarction lasting greater than 30 minutes but less than 12 hours. The patients also required electrocardiographic evidence of acute STEMI for inclusion, characterized as cumulative ST-segment elevation of at least 4 mm in at least 2 contiguous leads.

Who Was Excluded: Patients were excluded if they had a contraindication to fibrinolysis, left-bundle branch block, acute myocardial infarction and fibrinolysis within the previous 30 days, pulseless femoral arteries, previous coronary artery bypass surgery, renal failure, diabetes treated with metformin, non-ischemic heart disease, or a non-cardiac related life expectancy of less than 12 months. Patients were also excluded if they were high risk for transfer described as the presence of cardiogenic shock, persistent life-threatening arrhythmias, or need for mechanical ventilation.

How Many Patients: 1572 (1129 from referral hospitals and 443 from invasive-treatment centers)

Study Overview: See Figure 18.1 for an overview of the study design.

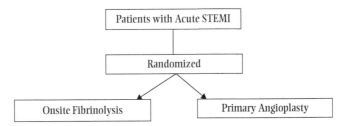

Figure 18.1 Summary of the DANAMI-2 trial design. The study consisted of two sub-studies, with randomization occurring at referral hospitals and invasive-treatment centers. Results were analyzed within the sub-studies separately, and combined.

Study Intervention: Patients in the fibrinolysis group received an oral aspirin, intravenous (IV) beta-blocker, IV tissue plasminogen activator (t-PA) bolus followed by an infusion, and an IV heparin bolus (5000 IU) followed by an infusion. In cases of failed reperfusion, reinfarction, or recurrent ischemia, patients underwent repeated fibrinolysis prior to rescue angioplasty.

Patients assigned to the angioplasty group received an oral aspirin, IV beta-blocker, and IV heparin bolus. Some patients received IIb/IIIa inhibitors at the discretion of the treating physician. Patients presenting to referral hospitals were transferred directly to the catheterization suite at the invasive-treatment center. Angioplasty was performed on the infarct-related artery if it was totally occluded, had a greater than 30% stenosis, or had a thrombolysis in myocardial infarction

(TIMI) grade flow of less than three. P2Y12 receptor inhibitors were administered for one month following stenting. In cases of recurrent ischemia, patients underwent repeat angioplasty.

Follow-Up: 30 days

Endpoints: Primary outcome: A composite of death from any cause, clinical reinfarction, or disabling stroke at follow-up.

RESULTS

The trial contained two concurrent substudies: patients enrolled at referral hospitals and patients enrolled at invasive-treatment centers. Results were analyzed for each substudy separately as well as for both substudies combined.

- In the angioplasty group, the median times from symptom onset to balloon inflation were 224 and 188 minutes for referral and invasive-treatment centers, respectively.
- The transfer time from referral hospitals for angioplasty (i.e., time from randomization to arrival at the catheterization suite) was less than 2 hours in 96% of patients with a median distance traveled of 50 kilometers (range of 3 to 150 km). The majority (64%) of these patients were within 50 km of invasive-treatment centers.
- Adverse events during transportation of patients to invasive-treatment centers were infrequent, with atrial fibrillation (2.5%), advanced heart block (2.3%), and ventricular fibrillation (1.4%) accounting for the most common events.
- Of the patients assigned to the fibrinolysis group, 99% received t-PA. Of the patients randomized to the angioplasty group, 98% underwent angiography, 87% underwent angioplasty, 80.7% underwent stenting, and 39.2% received GP IIb/IIIa inhibitors.
- Angioplasty was found superior to fibrinolysis with respect to the composite endpoint; however, when taken separately, a statistically significant reduction was achieved only with reinfarction, not with disabling stroke or death (see Figure 18.2). This was true with all hospitals combined, or when considering referral hospitals and invasive-treatment centers, separately.
- At 30 days of follow-up, coronary-artery bypass surgery or angioplasty was performed on 18.9% of patients in the fibrinolysis group. Repeat angioplasty or coronary-artery bypass surgery was performed on 9.1% of patients in the angioplasty group.

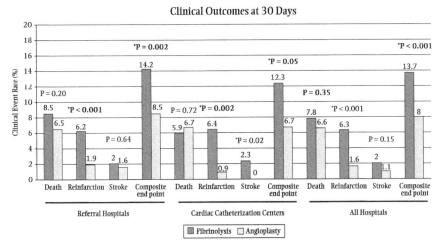

Figure 18.2 Summary of DANAMI-2's Key Findings. Clinical significance denoted by (*). Note, a statistically significant reduction was consistently achieved in re-infarction and the composite endpoint.

Criticisms and Limitations:

- Of the 4,278 patients that presented with STEMI and were screened for the study, only 37% were enrolled. Excluded patients were likely to have higher intervention-related complications and mortality, such as patients with history of diabetes, peripheral vascular disease, and prior coronary revascularization surgery. If these patients were included in the study, the difference in the composite endpoint between fibrinolysis and angioplasty groups may have been smaller. However, subsequent studies have suggested that higher-risk patients, such as those with hemodynamic instability, prior MI, or advanced age, may derive a greater benefit from percutaneous coronary intervention (PCI).[2]
- P2Y12 receptor inhibitors were administered for 30 days after stenting in 80.7% of patients in the angioplasty group. Because reinfarction is thought to proceed via a platelet-dependent mechanism, treatment with the P2Y12 receptor inhibitors may have provided additional benefit to patients in the angioplasty group. In a separate study, clopidogrel plus aspirin was shown to reduce myocardial infarction or death due to cardiovascular events in patients with unstable angina.[3] However, in a study similar to the DANAMI-2 trial evaluating fibrinolysis versus angioplasty at referral hospitals, a P2Y12 receptor inhibitor was included in both reperfusion strategies and provided results similar to the DANAMI-2 trial.[4]

- The efficacy of both fibrinolysis and angioplasty diminished with increasing time to implementation. The transfer time from referral hospitals for angioplasty in the DANAMI-2 trial was 2 hours or less in over 95% of the patients. For this study to be applicable, an infrastructure that allows similar transfer times to treatment centers must be present.

Other Relevant Studies and Information:

- Multiple studies have proven that fibrinolysis reduces infarct size, preserves left ventricular function, and decreases mortality in patients with STEMI; however, the benefit diminishes over time with negligible benefit 12 hours after symptom onset. There is no survival benefit of fibrinolytics in the setting of unstable angina (UA) or non-ST elevation myocardial infarction (NSTEMI).[5-6]
- Several randomized trials have validated that primary angioplasty is superior to fibrinolysis when therapy is administered within 12 hours of symptom onset.[7-8] A meta-analysis of these trials revealed a lower rate of death (5% vs. 7%), reinfarction (3% vs. 7%), and a composite endpoint of death, reinfarction, or stroke (8% vs. 14%).[8]
- Similar to the DANAMI-2 trial, other studies have compared immediate transfer for primary angioplasty versus onsite fibrinolysis for STEMI patients presenting to hospitals without cardiac catheterization capabilities.[1,4,9-11] A meta-analysis of these studies demonstrated significant reductions in reinfarction, stroke, and a composite endpoint (death, reinfarction, or stroke) when compared to fibrinolysis as well as a non-significant reduction in death.[8]
- A long-term follow-up study to the DANAMI-2 trial showed the benefit of primary angioplasty over fibrinolysis was maintained.[12] With a median follow-up of 7.8 years, a composite endpoint of death or reinfarction was significantly reduced with the primary angioplasty (35%) as opposed to fibrinolysis (44.3%) among patients from referral hospitals.
- For patients presenting to hospitals without PCI-capabilities, the 2013 ACC/AHA Guidelines for management of STEMI recommend immediate transfer to a PCI-capable facility when the anticipated time from first medical contact to balloon inflation is less than 120 minutes.[13] If this time is anticipated to be more than 120 minutes, fibrinolytic therapy should be administered if there are no contraindications. When indicated, fibrinolytics should be administered within 30 minutes of hospital arrival.

Summary and Implications: In patients presenting with STEMI and symptom duration of less than 12 hours, primary angioplasty is superior to fibrinolysis even when patients require transfer to facilities capable of cardiac catheterization, provided that transfer time (i.e., first medical contact to balloon time) is under 2 hours. Fibrinolysis is still recommended if the anticipated transfer time is greater than 2 hours and there are no contraindications.

CLINICAL CASE: ANGIOPLASTY VERSUS FIBRINOLYTICS IN ACUTE ST-ELEVATION MYOCARDIAL INFARCTION

Case History:
A 67-year-old male with hypertension and hyperlipidemia presents to a rural community emergency department with 3 hours of substernal chest pain. His blood pressure is 135/78, heart rate is 85, and oxygen saturation on room air is 97%. An EKG reveals 2-mm ST elevations in leads V1–4. A diagnosis of STEMI is made. Based upon the results of the DANAMI-2 trial, how should this patient be managed?

Suggested Answer:
For patients with STEMI presenting to hospitals without PCI capabilities, the DANAMI-2 trial demonstrated that primary angioplasty is preferred over fibrinolysis as the method of reperfusion given the time from first medical contact to balloon inflation is less than 2 hours. In addition, the trial verified that patients without cardiogenic shock, life-threatening arrhythmias, or a need for mechanical ventilation can be transferred safely with a low incidence of complications.

The patient in this vignette is typical of patients in the DANAMI-2 trial. If there is no onsite cardiac catheterization suite, he should be transferred to the nearest capable facility for PCI providing this can be accomplished within 2 hours of initial arrival. If this is not possible, a fibrinolytic agent should be administered within 30 minutes of initial arrival. In addition, the patient should receive an aspirin, beta-blocker, and oxygen. Nitroglycerin and morphine may also be helpful while awaiting initiation of reperfusion therapy. The decision to initiate anticoagulation or anti-platelet agents should be made in conjunction the cardiologist receiving the patient.

References
1. Andersen HR et al. A comparison of coronary angioplasty with fibrinolytic therapy in acute myocardial infarction. *N Engl J Med.* 2003;349(8):733–742.

2. Grines C et al. Primary coronary angioplasty compared with intravenous thrombo-lytic therapy for acute myocardial infarction: six-month follow up and analysis of individual patient data from randomized trials. *Am Heart J.* 2003;145:47–57.

3. Mehta SR et al. Effects of pretreatment with clopidogrel and aspirin followed by long-term therapy in patient undergoing percutaneous coronary intervention: the PCI-CURE study. *Lancet.* 2001;358:527–533.

4. Widimsky P et al. Multicentre randomized trial comparing transport to primary angioplasty vs immediate thrombolysis vs combined strategy for patients with acute myocardial infarction presenting to a community hospital without a catheterization laboratory: the PRAGUE study. *Eur Heart J.* 2000;21:823–831.

5. Gruppo Italiano per lo Studio della Streptochinasi nell'Infarto Miocardico (GISSI). Effectiveness of intravenous thrombolytic treatment in acute myocardial infarction. *Lancet.* 1986;1(8478):397–402.

6. Fibrinolytic Therapy Trialists' (FTT) Collaborative Group. Indications for fibrino-lytic therapy in suspected acute myocardial infarction: collaborative overview of early mortality and major morbidity results from all randomised trials of more than 1000 patients. *Lancet.* 1994;343(8893):311–322.

7. The Global Use of Strategies to Open Occluded Coronary Arteries in Acute Coronary Syndromes (GUSTO IIb) Angioplasty Substudy Investigators. A clinical trial comparing primary coronary angioplasty with tissue plasminogen activator for acute myocardial infarction. *N Engl J Med.* 1997;336(23):1621–1628.

8. Keeley EC et al. Primary angioplasty versus intravenous thrombolytic therapy for acute myocardial infarction: a quantitative review of 23 randomised trials. *Lancet.* 2003;361:13–20.

9. Widimsky P et al. Long distance transport for primary angioplasty vs immediate thrombolysis in acute myocardial infarction. Final results of the randomized national multicenter trial—PRAGUE-2. *Eur Heart J.* 2003;24(1):94–104.

10. Vermeer F et al. Prospective randomised comparison between thrombolysis, res-cue PTCA, and primary PRCA in patients with extensive myocardial infarction admitted to a hospital without PTCA facilities: a safety and feasibility study. *Heart.* 1999;82(4):426–431.

11. Grines CL et al. A randomized trial of transfer for primary angioplasty ver-sus on-site thrombolysis in patients with high-risk myocardial infarction: the Air Primary Angioplasty in Myocardial Infarction study. *J Am Coll Cardiol.* 2002;39(11)1713–1719.

12. Nielsen PH et al. Primary angioplasty versus fibrinolysis in acute myocardial infarction: long-term follow-up in the Danish acute myocardial infarction 2 trial. *Circulation.* 2010;121(13):1484–1491.

13. O'Gara PT et al. 2013 ACCF/AHA guideline for the management of ST-elevation myocardial infarction: executive summary: a report of the American College of Cardiology Foundation/American Heart Association Task Force on Practice Guidelines. *Circulation.* 2013;127:529–555.

Pulmonary, ARDS

19

The Acute Respiratory Distress Syndrome Network

Ventilation with Lower Tidal Volumes as Compared with Traditional Tidal Volumes for Acute Lung Injury and the Acute Respiratory Distress Syndrome

LALEH JALILIAN AND JEANINE WIENER-KRONISH

"In patients with acute lung injury and the acute respiratory distress syndrome, mechanical ventilation with a lower tidal volume than is traditionally used results in decreased mortality and increases the number of days without ventilator use."

—ARDS NETWORK ET AL.

Research Question: In patients with acute lung injury and the acute respiratory distress syndrome, does mechanical ventilation with a lower tidal volume improve clinical outcomes?[1]

Sponsor: National Heart, Blood, and Lung Institute

Year Study Began: 1996

Year Study Published: 2000

Study Location: 10 university centers of the Acute Respiratory Distress Syndrome Network of the National Heart, Lung, and Blood Institute

Who Was Studied: Patients receiving mechanical ventilation were eligible if they had an acute decrease in the ratio of partial pressure of arterial oxygen to fraction of inspired oxygen to 300 or less, bilateral pulmonary infiltrates on a chest x-ray consistent with the presence of edema, and no clinical evidence of left atrial hypertension, or (if measured) a pulmonary-capillary wedge pressure of 18 mm Hg or less.

Who Was Excluded: Patients were excluded if 36 hours had elapsed since they met the first three inclusion criteria; were younger than 18 years of age; were pregnant; had increased intracranial pressure, neuromuscular disease that could impair spontaneous breathing, sickle cell disease, or severe chronic respiratory disease; weighed more than 1 kg/cm of height; had burns over more than 30% of their body-surface area; had other conditions with an estimated 6-month mortality rate of more than 50%; had undergone bone marrow or lung transplantation; had chronic liver disease (as defined by Child–Pugh class C); or their attending physician refused.

How Many Patients: 861

Study Overview: Traditionally, patients receiving mechanical ventilation for acute lung injury (ALI) or acute respiratory distress syndrome (ARDS) requiring mechanical ventilation were subjected to high tidal volumes (10–15 mL/kg) in an effort to prevent atelectasis, maintain normal partial pressure of carbon dioxide and arterial pH (Figure 19.1). However, animal studies showed that higher tidal volumes were associated with increased lung injury. This multi-center, randomized, controlled trial compared traditional ventilation treatment, which involved an initial tidal volume of 12 mL/kg of predicted body weight and plateau pressure of 50 cm of water or less, with ventilation with a lower tidal volume of 6 mL/kg of predicted body weight and a plateau pressure of 30 cm of water or less.[1]

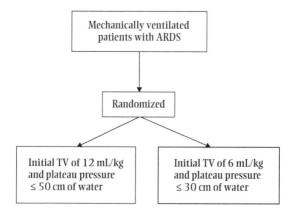

Figure 19.1 Summary of the study design.

Study Intervention: Patients were randomly assigned to receive mechanical ventilation involving either traditional tidal volumes or lower tidal volumes. Volume-assist–control mode was used for mechanical ventilation until either the patient was liberated from the device or for 28 days after randomization. In the lower tidal volume study group, the tidal volume was reduced to 6 mL/kg of predicted body weight within 4 hours after randomization and was subsequently reduced stepwise by 1 mL/kg of predicted body weight (to minimal tidal volume was 4 mL/kg of predicted body weight) if necessary to maintain plateau pressure at a level of no more than 30 cm of water. If plateau pressure fell below 25 cm of water, tidal volume was increased in steps of 1 mL/kg of predicted body weight until the plateau pressure was at least 25 cm of water or the tidal volume was 6 mL/kg of predicted body weight. If patients experienced severe dyspnea, the tidal volume could be increased to 7 to 8 mL/kg of predicted body weight if the plateau pressure remained at or below 30 cm of water.

In the traditional tidal volumes group, the initial tidal volume was 12 mL/kg of predicted body weight. This was subsequently reduced stepwise by 1 mL/kg of predicted body weight if necessary to maintain the plateau pressure at a level of ≤ 50 cm of water. The minimal tidal volume was 4 mL/kg of predicted body weight. If the plateau pressure decreased below 45 cm of water, the tidal volume was increased in steps of 1 mL/kg of predicted body weight until the plateau pressure was ≥ 45 cm of water or the tidal volume was 12 mL/kg of predicted body weight

Follow-Up: 180 days

Endpoints: The first primary outcome was death before a patient was discharged home and was breathing without assistance. The second primary outcome was the number of ventilator-free days from day 1 to day 28.

RESULTS

- The trial was stopped after an interim analysis of 861 patients revealed that mortality was lower in the lower tidal volume group than in the traditional tidal volume group (31.0% vs. 39.8%, $p = 0.007$). There was also a significant increase in the number of ventilator-free days in the low tidal volume group and in the number of days free from organ failure.
- The PEEP and FiO_2 were significantly higher in the lower tidal volume group and the P:F ratio was significantly lower on days 1 and 3. By day 7, PEEP and FiO_2 were significantly higher in the group treated with traditional tidal volumes.
- The respiratory rate was significantly higher in the lower tidal volume group on days 1 and 3, but minute ventilation was similar in the two

groups on these days. The $PaCO_2$ was significantly higher on days 1, 3, and 7, and arterial pH was significantly lower on days 1 and 3 in the group treated with lung protective ventilation.

- Plasma concentrations of Interleukin-6, which are a marker of systemic inflammation, were significantly lower in the low tidal volume group (Table 19.1).

Table 19.1. KEY FINDINGS FROM THE ARDS NET TRIAL

Variable	Group Receiving Lower Tidal Volumes	Group Receiving Traditional Tidal Volumes	P Value
Death before discharge home and breathing without assistance (%)	31.0	39.8	0.007
Breathing without assistance by day 28 (%)	65.7	55.0	< 0.001
No. of ventilator-free days, days 1 to 28	12	10	0.007
No. of days without failure of nonpulmonary organs or systems, days 1 to 28	15 +/− 11	12 +/− 11	0.006

Criticisms and Limitations:

- The trial was single blinded, as the clinicians caring for the patients were aware of the allocation arm. This may have resulted in differential treatment of patients in the two groups.
- The study was not simply a comparison of high and low tidal volumes, but rather a comparison of two distinct strategies of ventilatory management. Use of positive end-expiratory pressure (PEEP) was specified by the protocol, and the group treated with lower tidal volumes had significantly higher PEEP on days 1 and 3 of the study, than did the group treated with traditional tidal volumes. Since some evidence suggests that prevention of atelectasis, provided by PEEP, may be lung protective it is not possible in this study to determine whether it was the lower tidal volume, increased PEEP or combination of the two that actually had the beneficial effect on outcomes.
- The lower mortality rate in the group treated with lower tidal volumes was attributed to reduced ventilator-associated lung injury. However, information on the immediate causes of death is not provided. Since death may be attributable to extrapulmonary organ failure rather than

to the failure of pulmonary gas exchange, reduced lung injury may not sufficiently explain the improved outcome.

Other Relevant Studies and Information:

- An interesting finding from this study was that the lower tidal volume group actually had a lower mean PaO_2s than the control group, yet still resulted in improved mortality. This provides support for the theory that mortality in patients with ARDS does not typically result from inadequate oxygenation, but rather from extra pulmonary complications of ARDS.
- A lung-protective ventilation strategy is also potentially beneficial in patients who do not have ARDS at the onset of mechanical ventilation.[2] A recent meta-analysis showed that patients without ARDS ventilated with lower tidal volumes had a decreased lung injury development and mortality.[3]
- Recent guidelines for mechanical ventilation of severe ARDS recommend limitation of tidal volume (6 mL/kg predicted body weight), adequate high PEEP (>12 cm H_2O), a recruitment maneuver in special situations, and a "balanced" respiratory rate of 20–30/min.[4]

Summary and Implications: This study suggest that patients with ARDS had improved survival and a reduction in days of mechanical ventilation when a lung-protective ventilation strategy was employed. This strategy consisted of a reduction in tidal volume to 6 mL/kg of predicted weight, maintaining distending pressures ≤ 30 cm H_2O, and using PEEP to prevent atelectasis and support oxygenation. A lung-protective ventilation strategy may also be beneficial among mechanically ventilated patients without ARDS; however, further data are needed.

CLINICAL CASE: USING THE ARDS-NET STUDY

Case History:

A 45-year-old woman with predicted body weight of 50 kg has acute respiratory distress syndrome as a result of sepsis. She is currently being mechanically ventilated with TV 300 mL R 30 PEEP 8 40% FiO_2. Her peak pressure is 37 and plateau pressure is 34. Her most recent arterial blood gas is pH 7.31 PCO_2 44 and PO_2 80. Based on the ARDS-Net study, what is most appropriate next step in management of her ventilator settings?

Suggested Answer:

The ARDS Net Study demonstrated that a "lung protective" ventilation strategy consisting of low tidal volume, limitation of plateau pressure, and appropriate PEEP was associated with reduced mortality compared to conventional ventilation. While the tidal volume for the patient in the vignette is 6 mL/kg predicted body weight the plateau pressure is elevated. Based on the ARDS Net trial protocol when the plateau airway pressure is > 30 cm H_2O, the tidal volume should be decreased in 1 mL/kg PBW increments to a minimum of 4 mL/kg PBW. The respiratory rate will need to be increased (up to a maximum of 35 breaths/min) as the tidal volume is decreased, so that the ventilator continues to deliver the patient's entire minute ventilation. The plateau airway pressure should be checked at least every four hours and after each change in PEEP or tidal volume. The goal plateau airway pressure is ≤ 30 cm H_2O. A reasonable oxygenation goal during low tidal volume ventilation is an arterial oxygen tension (PaO_2) between 55 and 80 mm Hg. This is typically achieved by adjusting the fraction of inspired oxygen (FiO_2) and the applied PEEP. According to the ARDS Net protocol, a minimum PEEP of 5 cm H_2O should be used. Available evidence does not support the use of higher PEEP, compared to lower PEEP, in unselected patients with ARDS.

References

1. The Acute Respiratory Distress Syndrome Network: Ventilation with lower tidal volumes as compared with traditional tidal volumes for acute lung injury and the acute respiratory distress syndrome. *N Engl J Med.* 2000;342:1301–1308.
2. Fuller BM, Mohr NM, Drewry AM, Carpenter CR: Lower tidal volume at initiation of mechanical ventilation may reduce progression to acute respiratory distress syndrome: a systematic review. *Crit Care.* 2013;17: R11.
3. Serpa Neto A, Cardoso SO, Manetta JA, et al. Association between use of lung-protective ventilation with lower tidal volumes and clinical outcomes among patients without acute respiratory distress syndrome: a meta-analysis. *JAMA.* 2012;308:1651–1659.
4. Bein T, Grasso S, Moerer O, et al. The standard of care of patients with ARDS: ventilatory settings and rescue therapies for refractory hypoxemia. *Intensive Care Med.* 2016;42: 699–711.

20

Neuromuscular Blockers in Early Acute Respiratory Distress Syndrome

DUNCAN MCLEAN AND MATTHIAS EIKERMANN

"A brief period of paralysis early in the course of ARDS may facilitate lung-protective mechanical ventilation by improving patient– ventilator synchrony and allowing for the accurate adjustment of tidal volume and pressure levels . . . "

—PAPAZIAN ET AL.

Research Question: Do neuromuscular blocking agents (NMBs) improve outcomes in patients with acute respiratory distress syndrome who are receiving mechanical ventilation?[1]

Funding: Assistance Publique-Hôpitaux de Marseille, and Ministère de la Santé, France

Year Study Began: 2006

Year Study Published: 2010

Study Location: 20 ICUs in France

Who Was Studied: Patients who were endotracheally intubated and mechanically ventilated due to hypoxic respiratory failure, with a $PaO_2:FiO_2$ ratio < 150 and receiving PEEP of $\geq$ 5 cm H_2O and tidal volumes of 6–8 mL/kg of predicted body weight.

Who Was Excluded: Patients < 18 years old, with left atrial hypertension (pulmonary capillary wedge pressure ≥ 18 mm Hg, already receiving neuromuscular blockade at time of enrollment, known pregnancy, increased intracranial pressure, severe chronic respiratory disease requiring long-term oxygen therapy, actual body weight > 1 kg/cm of height, severe chronic liver disease, bone-marrow transplantation or chemotherapy-induced neutropenia, pneumothorax, expected duration of mechanical ventilation < 48 hours.

How Many Patients: 1326 patients assessed for eligibility, 986 excluded, 340 underwent randomization.

Study Overview: See Figure 20.1 for an overview of the study design.

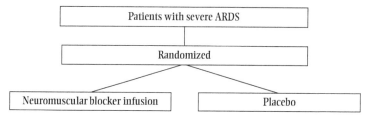

Figure 20.1 Summary of ACURASYS' study design.

Study Intervention: Sedation in both groups was titrated according to the Ramsay sedation scale. Patients received either a 15 mg bolus of cisatracurium followed by a 37.5 mg per hour cisatracurium infusion for 48 hours, or an identical volume of placebo. Cisatracurium and placebo solutions were prepared in identical vials by a study pharmacist.

Patients in either group who achieved plateau pressures of > 32 cm H_2O for over 10 minutes were allowed to be given an open-label bolus of 20 mg cisatracurium twice in 24-hours.

Follow-Up: 90 days

Endpoints: Primary outcome: 90-day mortality, Secondary outcomes: 28-day mortality, number of days outside the ICU, number of days without organ or system failure, barotrauma, ICU-acquired paresis, Medical Research Council scores* on day 28 and at time of ICU discharge and number of ventilator-free days.

---

* The scores are calculated from the Medical Research Council scale that assesses three muscle groups in each arm and leg. The score for each muscle group can range from 0 (paralysis) to 5 (normal strength), with the overall score ranging from 0 to 60.

RESULTS

- The crude 90-day mortality was 31.6% in the NMB infusion group versus 40.7% in the placebo group ($P = 0.08$). Mortality at 28 days was 23.7% in the cisatracurium vs. 33.3% in the placebo group ($P = 0.05$).
- After adjustment for both the baseline PaO_2:FIO_2 and plateau pressure and the Simplified Acute Physiology II score, the hazard ratio for death at 90 days in the cisatracurium group, as compared with the placebo group, was 0.68 ($P = 0.04$).
- The NMB group had more days off the ventilator, a greater number of days without extra-pulmonary organ failure and spent more days outside the ICU during the first 28-days.
- The NMB infusion group experienced less barotrauma (5.1% vs. 11.7%) and pneumothorax (4.0% vs. 11.7%) than the placebo group.
- There was no difference in ICU-acquired weakness as measured by MRC scores between groups (55% vs. 55%) at both day 28 and upon discharge from the ICU (Table 20.1).

Table 20.1. SUMMARY OF ACURASYS' KEY FINDINGS

Outcome	NMB group	Placebo group	P value
90-day mortality	31.6%	40.7%	0.08
28-day mortality	42.0%	54.0%	0.05
Number of days outside the ICU in first 90 days	47.7	39.5	0.03
Number of days without organ failure in first 28 days	15.8	12.2	0.01
Barotrauma	5.1%	11.7%	0.03
No ICU-acquired paresis at 28-days	70.8%	67.5%	0.64
Ventilator-free days in first 90 days	53.1	44.6	0.03

Criticisms and Limitations:

- Despite being described as "double-blind," patients not receiving NMBs would likely have triggered the ventilator, introducing the possibility that caregivers would not have remained blinded to study group allocation, therefore introducing bias.
- No information regarding managing patient-ventilator dyssynchrony was provided. It is possible that the poorer outcomes demonstrated in the placebo group were due to inadequate management of ventilator dyssynchrony. Other strategies exist to optimize ventilator synchrony and transpleural pressure, such as flow/time waveform analysis, sedation

titration, and adjustment of ventilator trigger thresholds and esophageal manometry.[2-4] These may achieve similarly improved outcomes without introducing the risk of NMBs such as worsened ICU-related weakness. The study did not assess the use of a neuromuscular blocking agent late in the course of ARDS or their use on the basis of plateau pressure or transpulmonary-pressure measurements. It is not known if later initiation of cisatracurium or titration based on respiratory parameters might provide benefit.

- Half of the patients in the placebo group received 1 dose of open-label cisatracurium—which is not common practice—raising questions about whether the comparator group reflected current practice.
- The study used a high fixed dose of cisatracurium not adjusted by use of train-of-4 stimulation, which differs from usual practice.

Other Relevant Studies and Information:

- Several small randomized studies have demonstrated reduced levels of inflammatory cytokines in patients receiving NMB infusions.[5,6]
- NMBs have been implicated in ICU-related weakness.[7,8]
- The use of NMBs in the operating room predicts post-operative pulmonary complications in a dose-dependent manner.[9,10]
- Rocuronium is associated with worsening of diaphragmatic weakness in the ICU.[11]
- The use of NMBs in the ICU is associated with PTSD after discharge.[12]
- Recent practice guidelines recommend that an NMB be administered by continuous IV infusion early in the course of ARDS for patients with a PaO_2/FiO_2 less than 150.[13]

Summary and Implications: Patients with severe ARDS may benefit from short-term NMB infusions, probably due to optimization of transpulmonary pressures, therefore making barotrauma less likely. These effects may also be achieved using other approaches to control the increased respiratory drive, such as opioid and sedative infusions, without some of the adverse effects of NMBs, such as immobilization. When using NMBs to temporarily immobilize the diaphragm, the clinician needs to conduct a risk-benefit assessment to balance the goal of lung protection while minimizing the harms.

CLINICAL CASE: NMBS IN ARDS

Case History:

A 57-year-old male develops systemic sepsis after major abdominal surgery. He is intubated and mechanically ventilated due to worsening hypoxia. Chest X-ray imaging demonstrates bilateral patchy infiltrates and blood gas analysis reveals a PaO_2:FiO_2 of 120. The ventilator is alarming due to high peak pressures and is unable to achieve 6 mL per kg tidal breaths. The ICU team is considering how to improve oxygenation while implementing a strategy to minimize ventilator-associated injury.

Based on the results of the ACURASYS trial, how should the ICU team proceed with ventilator management?

Suggested Management:

The patient in this vignette is demonstrating signs of severe ARDS, decreased lung compliance, and potential patient-ventilator dyssynchrony.

The ACURASYS trial demonstrated that patients with severe ARDS who are managed with NMB infusions experience decreased 28-day mortality and reduced ventilator-associated lung injury such as barotrauma.

ARDS may result from a wide range of precipitating pathologies, and critically ill patients vary in their disease burden. Therefore it is important to treat each case on an individual basis, making treatment decisions based upon an assessment of the risks and benefits. NMBs may improve outcomes by enhancing patient-ventilator synchrony and reducing oxygen consumption; however, alternative strategies—such as the use of sedative infusions—also exist, and these alternative strategies may be associated with fewer associated adverse effects.

References

1. Papazian L, Forel J-M, Gacouin A, et al. Neuromuscular blockers in early acute respiratory distress syndrome. *N Engl J Med.* 2010;363(12):1107–1116. doi:10.1056/NEJMoa1005372.
2. O'Gara B, Fan E, Talmor DS. Controversies in the management of severe ARDS: optimal ventilator management and use of rescue therapies. *Semin Respir Crit Care Med.* 2015;36(6):823–834. doi:10.1055/s-0035-1564889.
3. Mellott KG, Grap MJ, Munro CL, et al. Patient ventilator asynchrony in critically ill adults: Frequency and types. *Heart and Lung.* 2014;43(3):231–243. doi:10.1016/j.hrtlng.2014.02.002.
4. Mellott KG, Grap MJ, Munro CL, Sessler CN, Wetzel PA. Patient-ventilator dyssynchrony: clinical significance and implications for practice. *Critical Care Nurse.* 2009;29(6):41–55. doi:10.4037/ccn2009612.
5. Gainnier M, Roch A, Forel J-M, et al. Effect of neuromuscular blocking agents on gas exchange in patients presenting with acute respiratory distress syndrome. *Crit Care Med.* 2004;32(1):113–119. doi:10.1097/01.CCM.0000104114.72614.BC.
6. Forel J-M, Roch A, Marin V, et al. Neuromuscular blocking agents decrease inflammatory response in patients presenting with acute respiratory distress syndrome. *Crit Care Med.* 2006;34(11):2749–2757. doi:10.1097/01.CCM.0000239435.87433.0D.

7. Puthucheary Z, Rawal J, Ratnayake G, Harridge S, Montgomery H, Hart N. Neuromuscular blockade and skeletal muscle weakness in critically ill patients. *Am J Respir Crit Care Med.* 2012;185(9):911–917. doi:10.1164/rccm.201107-1320OE.

8. Kress JP, Hall JB. ICU-acquired weakness and recovery from critical illness. *N Engl J Med.* 2014;370(17):1626–1635. doi:10.1056/NEJMra1209390.

9. Grosse-Sundrup M, Henneman JP, Sandberg WS, et al. Intermediate acting non-depolarizing neuromuscular blocking agents and risk of postoperative respiratory complications: prospective propensity score matched cohort study. *BMJ.* 2012;345(oct15 5):e6329–e6329. doi:10.1136/bmj.e6329.

10. McLean DJ, Diaz-Gil D, Farhan HN, Ladha KS, Kurth T, Eikermann M. Dose-dependent Association between Intermediate-acting neuromuscular-blocking agents and postoperative respiratory complications. *Anesthesiology.* 2015;122(6):1201–13. doi:10.1097/ALN.0000000000000674.

11. Eikermann M. Muscle weakness after administration of neuromuscular blocking agents: Do not immobilize the diaphragm unnecessarily. *Crit Care Med.* 2007;35(6):1634–35. doi:10.1097/01.CCM.0000266804.62808.2B.

12. Nelson BJ, Weinert CR, Bury CL, Marinelli WA, Gross CR. Intensive care unit drug use and subsequent quality of life in acute lung injury patients. *Crit Care Med.* 2000;28(11):3626–3630.

13. Murray MJ, DeBlock H, Erstad B, et al. Clinical practice guidelines for sustained neuromuscular blockade in the adult critically ill patient. *Crit Care Med.* 2016 Nov;44(11):2079–2103.

21

Prone Positioning in Severe Acute Respiratory Distress Syndrome

The PROSEVA Trial

ANDREA COPPADORO AND GUISEPPE FOTI

We randomly assigned 466 patients with severe ARDS ($PaO_2/FiO_2 < 150$ mm Hg) to undergo prone-positioning sessions of at least 16 hours or to be left in the supine position. The 28-day mortality was 16.0% in the prone group and 32.8% in the supine group (P<0.001). [. . .] In patients with severe ARDS, early application of prolonged prone-positioning sessions significantly decreased 28-day and 90-day mortality.
                                                                —GUÉRIN ET AL.

Research Question: Does the early application of prone positioning improve survival in patients with moderate/severe acute respiratory distress syndrome (ARDS)?[1]

Sponsor: Programme Hospitalier de Recherche Clinique National 2006 and 2010 of the French Ministry of Health

Year Study Began: 2008

Year Study Published: 2013

Study Location: 26 ICUs in France and 1 in Spain, which used prone positioning in daily practice for more than 5 years

Who Was Studied: Critically ill adult patients with respiratory failure requiring mechanical ventilation for severe ARDS. Severe ARDS was defined as an arterial partial pressure of oxygen/fraction of inspired oxygen (PaO_2/FiO_2) ratio < 150 mm Hg, an FiO_2 ≥0.6, a positive end-expiratory pressure of at least 5 cm of water, and a tidal volume of 6 mL per kilogram of predicted body weight.

Who Was Excluded: Patients with elevated intracranial pressure, hemoptysis, recent tracheal surgery, recent facial trauma or facial surgery, DVT treated for < 2 days, recent cardiac pacemaker insertion, unstable spine, femur, or pelvic fractures, hypotension, pregnancy, single anterior chest tube with air leaks, use of inhaled nitric oxide or almitrine bismesylate use before inclusion, ECMO before inclusion, lung transplantation, burns > 20% TBSA, NIV delivered for more than 24 hours before inclusion, life expectancy of less than one year. Patients quickly improving during the 12–24 hours stabilization period were also excluded.

How Many Patients: 1434 were screened; 576 were eligible, and 466 patients were included. About one-hundred eligible patients were excluded.

Study Overview: This multicenter clinical trial was designed to determine whether prone positioning has any beneficial effects in ARDS patients with severe hypoxemia when initiated within 24 hours after onset of ARDS and sustained for longer duration of at least 16 hours per day (Figure 21.1).

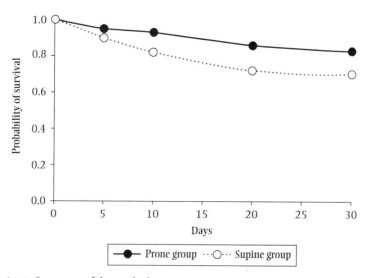

Figure 21.1 Summary of the study design.

Study Intervention: After a stabilization period of 12 to 24 hours, patients assigned to the prone group were immediately turned to the prone position, and kept prone for sessions of at least 16 hours per day until day 28 (Figure 21.1). The criteria for discontinuing prone treatment included oxygenation improvement persisting during supine sessions; worsening of the PaO_2/FiO_2 ratio in the prone position; and the occurrence of complications such as nonscheduled extubation, main-stem bronchus intubation, endotracheal-tube obstruction, hemoptysis, cardiac arrest, or hypotension lasting for more than 5 minutes

Mechanical ventilation was modeled after the "lung protective" ARDSNet protocol, with tidal volume targeted at 6 mL per kilogram predicted body weight, PEEP level selected from a PEEP–FiO_2 table, end-inspiratory plateau pressure goal ≤30 cm H_2O and goal pH 7.20–7.45. Physiological variables were measured at predetermined times in both groups.

Follow-Up: 90 days.

Endpoints: Primary endpoint: Mortality at day 28. *Secondary end points*: Mortality at day 90, rate and time to successful extubation, tracheostomy rate, ICU length of stay, complications, use of noninvasive ventilation, the number of days free from organ dysfunction; respiratory system mechanics, ventilator settings and arterial blood gas during the first week after randomization.

RESULTS

- The 28-day mortality was significantly lower in the prone group than in the supine group: 16.0% versus 32.8% ($P < 0.001$).
- The mean number of ventilator free days was greater in the prone group than in the supine group: 14 versus 10 ($P < 0.001$).
- The incidence of complications did not differ significantly between the groups, except for the incidence of cardiac arrests, which occurred more frequently in the supine group (Table 21.1).

Table 21.1. OUTCOMES FROM THE PROSEVA STUDY

	Supine Group (N = 229)	Prone Group (N = 237)	P Value
Mortality—no. (% [95% CI])			
At day 28	32.8 [26.4–38.6]	16.0 [11.3–20.7]	<0.001
At day 90	41.0 [34.6–47.4]	23.6 [18.2–29.0]	<0.001
Length of ICU stay, assessed at day 90—days			
Survivors	26±27	24 ± 22	0.05
Nonsurvivors	18±15	21 ± 20	
28 day ventilation-free days	10±10	14 ± 9	<0.001
Cardiac arrest (%)	31	16	0.02

Criticisms and Limitations:

- The trial involved a highly select group of patients with less than one third of screened patients with ARDS undergoing randomization, and 60% ineligible on the basis of exclusion criteria.
- There were imbalances in baseline characteristics between the two groups, with more severely ill patients enrolled in the control group, as evidenced by higher Sequential Organ Failure Assessment scores and increased vasopressor requirements, compared with the PPV group. This difference between the groups could have biased the result toward benefit for the PPV group.
- Blinding was impossible and may have resulted in differences in care received by the two groups.
- It has been suggested that the positive effects obtained by prone positioning could also be obtained by setting high PEEP levels. Currently no data are available comparing the effects of prone positioning versus high PEEP levels.[2]
- Management of the prone patient is technically challenging and requires training. The study was conducted in centers where practitioners are highly skilled and trained in prone ventilation. Therefore results may not be generalizable to centers with limited experience in prone positioning

Other Relevant Studies and Information:

- The first report on prone positioning in patients with ARDS appeared more than 40 years ago and described striking improvement of oxygenation when patients were turned from the supine to the prone position.[3]
- Over the last 15 years, five major trials have compared the prone and supine positions on survival in patients with ARDS. This sequence of trials enrolled patients who were progressively more hypoxemic; extended the duration of proning from 8 to more than 16 hours/ day; and more rigorously applied lung-protective ventilation. While meta-analyses incorporating data from the first four major trials showed significant survival benefit in patients with severe ARDS, the PROSEVA trial was the first study to confirm these benefits in a formal randomized study.
- Post-hoc analysis of data from the PROSEVA trial found that the improvement in survival with prone ventilation seen in patients with ARDS does not depend on whether the change in position improves gas exchange.[4] Rather it has been postulated that prone positioning protects

against ventilator induced lung injury by distributing stress and strain more homogeneously through the lung parenchyma.
- An ancillary study conducted in conjunction with the PROSEVA trial found that the occurrence of pressure ulcers was increased in patients who undergo prone positioning compared with supine positioning.[5]
- While these beneficial effects of prone positioning appear to confer a survival advantage in patients with severe forms of ARDS, its long-term use may not be effective for mild/moderate ARDS (PaO_2/FiO_2 greater than 150 mm Hg), as it may expose the patient to unnecessary risk of complications in the absence of proven benefits.[6]
- The Surviving Sepsis Guidelines recommend the prone position in adult patients with sepsis-induced ARDS and a PaO_2/FIO_2 ratio < 150.[7]

Summary and Implications: The PROSEVA trial found that for patients with ARDS and severe hypoxemia (PaO_2/FiO_2 < 150 mm Hg) persisting after a 12–24 hour stabilization period, prone positioning reduces mortality rates, provided well trained staff is available to implement this therapy. To be most effective, prone positioning should be performed at least 16 hours a day.

CLINICAL CASE: PRONE POSITIONING A PATIENT WITH SEVERE ARDS

Case History:
A 67-year-old man is admitted to the ICU with respiratory failure due to pneumonia. After intubation, initial ventilator settings are: tidal volume of 6 mL/kg, PEEP 12 cmH$_2$O and respiratory rate of 33 breaths/min. However, his oxygenation is severely compromised with a PaO_2/FiO_2 ratio 104; pCO$_2$ is 58 mm Hg and pH 7.27. Based on the results of this study, should you prone the patient?

Suggested Answer:
This study suggests that the use of prone positioning for patients with severe ARDS patients leads to reduced mortality if (1) performed in medical centers with experience with prone positioning, (2) started early (12–24 hours stabilization period), and (3) proning sessions are performed for at least 16 hours. The first priority is to stabilize the patient, collect data to confirm the diagnosis, and start the appropriate therapy. Use of neuromuscular blocking agents and the use of recruitment maneuvers may be beneficial in improving oxygenation. After patient stabilization, prone positioning should be considered, assuming trained staff is available on site.

References

1. Guérin C, Reignier J, Richard JC, et al. (PROSEVA Study Group). Prone positioning in severe acute respiratory distress syndrome. *N Engl J Med.* 2013; 368(23):2159–2168.
2. Beitler JR, Guérin C, Ayzac L, et al. PEEP titration during prone positioning for acute respiratory distress syndrome. *Crit Care.* 2015;19:436.
3. Piehl MA, Brown RS. Use of extreme position changes in acute respiratory failure. *Crit Care Med.* 1976;4:13–14.
4. Albert RK, Keniston A, Baboi L, Ayzac L, Guérin C, Proseva Investigators. Prone position-induced improvement in gas exchange does not predict improved survival in the acute respiratory distress syndrome. *Am J Respir Crit Care Med.* 2014;189(4):494–496.
5. Girard R, Baboi L, Ayzac L, Richard JC, Guérin C; Proseva trial group. The impact of patient positioning on pressure ulcers in patients with severe ARDS: results from a multicentre randomised controlled trial on prone positioning. *Intensive Care Med.* 2014;40(3):397–403.
6. Gattinoni L, Taccone P, Carlesso E, Marini JJ. Prone position in acute respiratory distress syndrome. Rationale, indications, and limits. *Am J Respir Crit Care Med.* 2013;188(11):1286–1293.
7. Rhodes A, Evans LE, Alhazzani W, et al. Surviving sepsis campaign: international guidelines for management of sepsis and septic shock: 2016. *Crit Care Med.* 2017;45(3):486–552.

Efficacy and Economic Assessment of Conventional Ventilatory Support versus Extracorporeal Membrane Oxygenation for Severe Adult Respiratory Failure (CESAR)

A Multicentre Randomized Controlled Trial

MATTHEW SIGAKIS

" . . . transferring of adult patients with severe but potentially reversible respiratory failure, whose Murray score exceeds 3.0 or who have a pH of less than 7.20 on optimum conventional management, to a centre with an ECMO-based management protocol to significantly improve survival without severe disability."

—PEEK GJ, ET AL.

Research Question: Does ECMO referral improve survival without severe disability in adult patients with severe respiratory failure? Is ECMO cost-effective compared to conventional ventilator support?[1]

Funding: United Kingdom National Health Service Technology Assessment, English National Specialist Commissioning Advisory Group, Scottish Department of Health, and Welsh Department of Health.

Year Study Began: 2001

Year Study Published: 2009

Study Location: A single ECMO center, Glenfield Hospital, and 92 conventional treatment centers and 11 referral hospitals in the United Kingdom.

Who Was Studied: Adults aged 18–65 years with severe but potentially reversible respiratory failure who also had either a (1) Murray score of ≥ 3.0 or (2) uncompensated hypercapnia (pH < 7.20). The Murray score is composed of four components: (1) chest radiograph; (2) hypoxemia score; (3) PEEP; and (4) static compliance of respiratory system. Reversibility was based on the clinical opinion of one of three on-duty ECMO consultants.

Who Was Excluded: (1) Patients maintained on high pressure (peak inspiratory pressure > 30 cm H_2O) or high fraction of inspired oxygen (> 0.80) ventilation for more than 7 days; (2) signs of intracranial bleeding; (3) contraindication to heparinization; (4) contraindication to continuation of active treatment.

How Many Patients: 766 patients were screened; 180 were enrolled.

Study Overview: See Figure 22.1 for an overview of the study design.

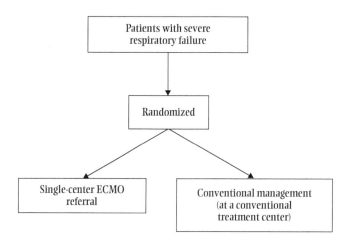

Figure 22.1 Summary of the study design.

Study Intervention: Patients in the extracorporeal membrane oxygenation (ECMO) referral group were transferred to a single center. If the patient was hemodynamically stable a standard protocol was used which consisted of pressure-controlled ventilation at Plateau Pressure ≤ 30 cm H_2O, positive end expiratory pressure titrated to optimum SaO_2, and FiO_2 titrated to maintain SaO_2 at more than 90%. In addition, diuretics were administered to achieve dry weight, target packed cell volume of 40%, prone positioning, and full nutrition were provided. If the patients did not respond to this protocol within 12 hours or were hemo-dynamically unstable, they received cannulation and ECMO. ECMO was veno-venous via cannulation of the femoral and right jugular veins. Ventilator settings were reduced gradually to allow lung rest (peak inspiratory pressure 20–25, positive end expiratory pressure 10–15, rate 10, and FiO_2 0.3). ECMO was continued until lung recovery, or until irreversible multiorgan failure.

Patients in the conventional management group received the "best critical care practice available in their center." While a specific management protocol was not mandated, treatment centers were advised to use a low-volume low-pressure ventilation strategy—i.e., tidal volume of 4–8 mL/kg bodyweight—and pressure plateau of less than 30 cm H_2O was recommended. Patients could not cross over to receive ECMO.

Follow-Up: 6 months

Endpoints: The primary outcome measured was death or severe disability at 6 months. Severe disability was defined as confinement to bed and inability to wash or dress alone.

Secondary outcomes included duration of ventilation, use of high-frequency oscillation or jet ventilation, use of nitric oxide, prone positioning, steroid use, ICU length of stay, and hospital length of stay. Additional outcomes measured in the ECMO referral group included method of ECMO (Veno-Venous or Veno-Arterial), duration of ECMO, blood flow, and sweep flow.

RESULTS

- 24% patients randomized to ECMO did not receive ECMO because they improved with conventional management (18%), died prior to or during transfer (5%), or had a contra-indication to heparin (1%). All patients assigned to conventional management received conventional management, although one conventional patient also received Arterio-Venous Extracorporeal CO_2 removal in a direct protocol violation. This patient survived and was analyzed according to the intention to treat as a conventional survivor.
- Survival without severe disability at 6 months was higher in the ECMO referral group compared with conventional management group (63% vs. 47%; $P = 0.03$).
- Cause of death in the ECMO referral group was most commonly multi-organ failure (42%) whereas cause of death in the conventional management group was more often due to respiratory failure (60%).
- ICU and hospital length of stay was longer in the ECMO referral group compared to the conventional management group.

- Mean healthcare costs per patient were higher for treatment of patients in the ECMO referral group compared with the conventional management group with a difference in costs of $65,519 in US dollars.

Criticisms and Limitations:

- Although the multiple centers provided conventional treatment only one (expert, high volume) center provided ECMO which raises the question of whether the results would be similar in smaller or less experienced centers. The conventional ventilation arm did not have a standardized protocol and only 70% of the control group were ventilated by low-tidal-volume and low-pressure ventilation according to the (ARDS) Network protocol. The absence of a strict lung protection protocol for the control group will undoubtedly have affected survival and although the ECMO group was compared to the care considered standard in the UK at the time the study raises the question of whether the conventional care was of an appropriate standard.
- Only two serious adverse events (SAEs) were described anecdotally in the ECMO group which is surprising, since recent ECMO studies report an incidence of severe adverse events ranging from 24% to 55%.[2] This raises questions of whether there was an underreporting of SAEs or a difference in the definition of SAEs compared with other studies.
- A number of new promising techniques for extracorporeal lung support have been developed in recent years, yet the study used "traditional" ECMO with roller pumps and high anticoagulation which were state of the art at the time.[3, 4] Future studies are needed to determine whether these ECMO advances will have a further benefit on survival.

Other Relevant Studies and Information:

- A cohort study of patients with severe influenza H1N1-related ARDS found that referral and transfer to an ECMO center was associated with lower hospital mortality (23.7 versus 52.5%).[5] Eighty five percent of the patients referred to an ECMO center received ECMO, while others improved with conventional ventilation.
- A retrospective multicenter review of data from the Extracorporeal Life Support Organization (ELSO) registry evaluated survival of adult ECMO respiratory failure patients during the period of 1986–2006. Of 1,473 patients, 50% survived to discharge.[6]

- A recent Cochrane systematic review was performed to determine whether use of veno-venous (VV) or venous-arterial (VA) ECMO in adults is more effective in improving survival compared with conventional respiratory and cardiac support.[7] Only four randomized controlled trials were identified that compared the intervention versus conventional treatment. The authors conclude that data on use of ECMO in patients with acute respiratory failure remain inconclusive given (1) the evidence to date (as of August, 2014) and (2) that patient treatment and practice with ECMO have considerably changed over time.
- The Extracorporeal Life Support Organization (ELSO) guidelines for adult respiratory failure recommend that ECMO should be considered when the risk of mortality is ≥ 50%, and is indicated when the risk of mortality ≥ 80%. ECMO is also indicated with CO_2 retention on mechanical ventilation despite high plateau pressures, severe air leak syndromes, need for intubation in a patient on lung transplant list, or for immediate cardiac or respiratory collapse.[8]

Summary and Implications: The CESAR trial results indicate that patients with severe but potentially reversible respiratory failure have improved survival without severe disability when transferred to a high volume center with expertise in ECMO. Although survival without severe disability was improved, it was at a significantly increased cost and length of hospital stay. Concerns regarding the generalizability of the findings warrant further investigation.

CLINICAL CASE: USING THE CESAR TRIAL

Case History:

A 47-year-old man previously healthy main is admitted to your ICU with respiratory failure from community-acquired pneumococcal pneumonia. He is intubated and is initiated on mechanical ventilation using the ARDSNet protocol. Over the next two days, he develops increased oxygen requirements and bilateral opacification on chest xray. His oxygenation worsens with partial pressure of oxygen (PaO_2) decreasing to 40 mm Hg, despite ventilatory support with a fraction of inspired oxygen (FIO_2) of 1.0 and a positive end-expiratory pressure (PEEP) of 20 cm of water. A neuromuscular blocking agent is administered, and he is placed in the prone position without improvement in his PaO_2. He remains hemodynamically stable without evidence of other end organ dysfunction. Your hospital does not offer ECMO. Based on the results of the CESAR trial, how should this patient be managed?

Suggested Answer:

The CESAR trial and other recent observational studies suggest that patients with severe but potentially reversible respiratory failure have improved survival when transferred to a center with an ECMO-based management protocol. The patient in the vignette has refractory hypoxemia despite maximal conventional therapy. Consultation and referral to an ECMO center should be considered.

References

1. Peek GJ, Mugford M, Tiruvoipati R, et al. Efficacy and economic assessment of conventional ventilatory support versus extracorporeal membrane oxygenation for severe adult respiratory failure (CESAR): a multicentre randomised controlled trial. *Lancet.* 2009;374(9698):1351–1363.
2. Hemmilla M, Rowe S, Boules TN, et al. Extracorporeal life support for severe acute respiratory distress syndrome in adults. *Ann Surg.* 2004;240: 595–607.
3. Bein T, Weber F, Philipp A, et al. A new pumpless extracorporeal interventional lung assist in critical hypoxemia/hypercapnia. *Crit Care Med.* 2006; 34: 1372–1377.
4. Floerchinger B, Philipp A, Foltan M, et al. Switch from venoarterial extracorporeal membrane oxygenation to arteriovenous pumpless extracorporeal lung assist. *Ann Thorac Surg.* 2010;89(1):125–131.
5. Noah MA, Peek GJ, Finney SJ, et al. Referral to an extracorporeal membrane oxygenation center and mortality among patients with severe 2009 influenza A(H1N1). *JAMA.* 2011; 306:1659.
6. Brogan TV, Thiagarajan RR, Rycus PT, et al. Extracorporeal membrane oxygenation in adults with severe respiratory failure: a multi-center database. Intensive *Care Med.* 2009; 35:2105.
7. Tramm R, Ilic D, Davies AR, et al. Extracorporeal membrane oxygenation for critically ill adults. *Cochrane Database Syst Rev.* 2015 Jan 22;1:CD010381.
8. Extracorporeal Life Support Organization (ELSO) Guidelines for Adult Respiratory Failure (2013). https://www.elso.org/Portals/0/IGD/Archive/FileManager/ 989d4d4d14 cusersshyerdocumentselsoguidelinesforadultrespiratory failure1.3.pdf. Last accessed 3/12/2017

Comparison of Two Fluid-Management Strategies in Acute Lung Injury

The FACTT Trial

ROSS GAUDET AND REBECCA KALMAN

"We developed a randomized study to compare conservative and liberal strategy of fluid management using explicit protocols in patients with acute lung injury. Although there was no significant difference in primary outcome of 60-day mortality, the conservative strategy of fluid management improved lung function and shortened the duration of mechanical ventilation and intensive care without increasing nonpulmonary-organ failures. These results support the use of a conservative strategy of fluid management."

—WIEDEMANN ET AL.

Research Question: Does a conservative versus liberal fluid-management protocol reduce death from any cause at 60 days in patients with acute lung injury?[1]

Sponsor: The National Heart, Lung, and Blood Institute Acute Respiratory Distress Syndrome (ARDS) Clinical Trials Network

Year Study Began: 2000

Year Study Published: 2006

Study Location: 20 North American hospitals

Who Was Studied: Patients who were intubated, received positive pressure ventilation, had a PaO_2/FiO_2 ratio of less than 300, and had bilateral infiltrates on chest x-ray without evidence of left atrial hypertension.

Who Was Excluded: Exclusion criteria included the presence of pulmonary-artery catheter after onset of acute lung injury; the presence of lung injury for > 48 hours; the inability to consent; the presence of comorbidities that would independently influence survival, ventilator weaning, or protocol compliance; and irreversible conditions where the estimated 6 month mortality rate was > 50%.

How Many Patients: 1,001

Study Overview: See Figure 23.1 for an overview of the study design.

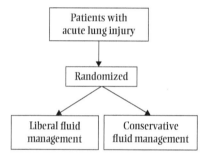

Figure 23.1 Summary of the study design.

Study Intervention: Patients were randomized in a 2 x 2 design to either conservative versus liberal fluid management strategy and to receive either a pulmonary artery-catheter (PAC) or a central venous catheter (CVC). For patients in both fluid management groups, ventilation was begun using the ARDSNet protocol within 1 hour after randomization and catheterization with either a pulmonary artery catheter or a central venous catheter was performed within 4 hours.

At least every 4 hours, patients were assigned to 1 of 20 protocol cells on the basis of 4 variables:

- Central venous pressure (CVP) or pulmonary-artery occlusion pressure (PAOP), depending on catheter assignment
- The presence or absence of shock (defined as a mean arterial pressure < 60 mm Hg or the need for a vasopressor [except for dopamine of ≤ 5 µg /kg/min])

- The presence or absence of oliguria (defined by a urinary output
  < 0.5 mL/kg/hr).
- The presence or absence of ineffective circulation (defined by a
  cardiac index < 2.5 liters/minute/meter^2 in the PAC group and by
  cold, mottled skin with a capillary-refilling time > 2 seconds in the
  CVC group).

Each cell is associated with an intervention and a reassessment interval.

For fluid boluses, clinicians were free to select isotonic crystalloid, albumin, or blood products, although the protocol dictated the volume of each administered.

If patients were in shock, treatment was left to the judgment of the physician until blood pressure stabilized, when vasopressor weaning was conducted according to the protocol.

Follow-Up: 60 days

Endpoints: Primary: death at 60 days. Secondary: ventilator-free days, ICU-free days, organ failure–free days, need for dialysis

RESULTS

- There was no significant difference in the primary outcome of
  mortality after 60 days between the two groups (conservative 25.5% vs.
  liberal 28.4%)
- The conservative fluid management group had 2.5 more
  ventilator-free days, 2.2 more ICU-free days than the liberal fluid
  management group.
- There were no significant differences in either the percentage of patients
  receiving renal-replacement therapy (conservative 10% vs. liberal 14%)
  or the average number of days of renal support.
- There were no significant interactions between baseline shock status
  and treatment with respect to the mortality rate or the number of
  ventilator-free days or ICU-free days (Table 23.1).

Table 23.1. SUMMARY OF THE STUDY'S KEY FINDINGS

Outcome	Conservative Strategy	Liberal Strategy	P-value
Mortality at 60 days	25.5%	28.4%	0.30
Ventilator-free days	14.6	12.1	< 0.001
ICU-free days	13.4	11.2	< 0.001
Patients requiring dialysis	10%	14%	0.06

Criticisms and Limitations:

- The trial's major design limitation was inability to blind clinicians or patients, which may have introduced bias. However, internal review of protocol adherence should have ameliorated this somewhat.
- The enrolled patients were relatively young (mean age 50 years), with mild disease severity. As a result, the generalizability of the findings may be limited.
- There was a delay of 24 hours after the establishment of acute lung injury before the study intervention was initiated. It is possible the results would have been different had the intervention been initiated immediately.
- The 7-day cumulative fluid balance was −136 ± 491 mL in the conservative-strategy group versus 6992 ± 502 mL in the liberal-strategy group. Therefore this was a study of even versus positive fluid balance. It is possible that a larger negative fluid balance may have resulted in better outcomes.[2]
- The trial may have been underpowered to detect differences in secondary outcomes between groups.

Other Relevant Studies and Information:

- A post hoc analysis of surgical patients enrolled in the FACTT had similar results with regard to the primary outcome: the risk of death did not vary with fluid management or catheter type. The conservative strategy resulted in one more ventilator-free day and ICU-free day in this subgroup.[3]
- A simplified conservative fluid protocol, "FACTT Lyte," may be just as effective as the more complex FACTT protocol.[4]
- Other mechanisms proposed to decrease pulmonary edema in ARDS include modulation of oncotic pressure with albumin administration and stimulation of active water transport from the alveoli.[5,6] Although albumin treatment has been suggested to improve oxygenation transiently in ARDS patients, insufficient evidence exists to justify its use.[7]
- The 2016 Surviving Sepsis guidelines recommend "a conservative fluid strategy for patients with established sepsis-induced ARDS who do not have evidence of tissue hypoperfusion."[8]

Summary and Implications: Conservative fluid management in patients with acute lung injury, with a goal of central venous pressure > 13 or pulmonary-artery occlusion pressure > 18, had a similar profile with respect to adverse events as did a liberal fluid management with a goal CVP > 18 or PAOP > 24. The conservative fluid strategy did, however, improve lung function and shortened the duration of mechanical ventilation and intensive care length of stay. These results support the use of a conservative strategy of fluid management in patients with acute lung injury.

CLINICAL CASE: COMPARISON OF TWO FLUID MANAGEMENT STRATEGIES IN ACUTE LUNG INJURY

Case History:

You are managing a patient with abdominal sepsis after undergoing a subtotal colectomy for perforated diverticulitis. For the past 2 days he has remained intubated and has been treated for abdominal sepsis with fluid resuscitation, vasopressors, and antibiotic therapy. He is no longer requiring vasopressor support but now has worsening oxygenation with PaO_2: FiO_2 ratio of 210 and bilateral infiltrates on chest film. Serum BUN and Creatinine are 24 and 1.7, which are unchanged from ICU admission. Bedside ultrasound reveals normal cardiac function and evidence of adequate fluid resuscitation. One of your colleagues suggests that in addition to maintaining a lung-protective ventilation strategy, you should insert a pulmonary artery catheter to guide your fluid management and avoid diuretics in order to prevent worsening kidney injury. How do you respond?

Suggested Answer:

This study suggests that implementation of a conservative fluid management protocol would decrease the length mechanical ventilation and ICU stay without increasing the potential for renal dysfunction or other end organ damage. A more appropriate fluid management strategy would be to administer diuretics aiming for a net zero fluid balance over the next week while continuing to monitor for evidence of end organ hypoperfusion. Insertion of a pulmonary artery catheter is unlikely to provide benefit.

References

1. Wiedemann H. et al. Comparison of two fluid-management strategies in acute lung injury. *N Engl J Med*. 2006;54:2564–2575.
2. Schuller D, Schuster D. Fluid-management strategies in acute lung injury. *N Engl J Med*. 2006;355:1175–1176.
3. Stewart SM, et al. Less is more: improved outcomes in surgical patients with conservative fluid administration and central venous catheter monitoring. *J Am Coll Surg*. 2009 May;208(5):725–733.

4. Grissom CK, et al. Fluid management with a simplified conservative protocol for the acute respiratory distress syndrome. *Crit Care Med.* 2015;43(2):288–295.

5. Perkins GD, McAuley DF, Thickett DR, Gao F. The beta-agonist lung injury trial (BALTI): a randomized placebo-controlled clinical trial. *Am J Respir Crit Care Med.* 2006;173:281–287.

6. Roch A, Guervilly C, Papazian L. Fluid management in acute lung injury and ARDS. *Ann Intensive Care.* 2011;1(1):16.

7. Uhlig C, Silva PL, Deckert S, Schmitt J, de Abreu MG. Albumin versus crystalloid solutions in patients with the acute respiratory distress syndrome: a systematic review and meta-analysis. *Crit Care.* 2014;18:R10.

8. Rhodes A, Evans LE, Alhazzani W, et al. Surviving Sepsis Campaign: International Guidelines for Management of Sepsis and Septic Shock: 2016. *Crit Care Med.* 2017;45(3):486–552.

Positive End-Expiratory Pressure Setting in Adults with ALI and ARDS

The ExPress Trial

J. AARON SCOTT AND VIVEK MOITRA

"A strategy for setting PEEP aimed at increasing alveolar recruitment while limiting hyperinflation did not significantly reduce mortality. However, it did improve lung function and reduce the duration of mechanical ventilation and the duration of organ failure."

—THE EXPRESS INVESTIGATORS

Research Question: Does targeting increased alveolar recruitment with PEEP in ALI/ARDS provide a mortality benefit?[1]

Funding: Centre Hospitalier Universitaire d'Angers, Ministere de la santé, and Association National pour le Traitement à Domicile de L'Insuffisance Respiratoire (ANTADIR)

Year Study Began: 2002

Year Study Published: 2008

Study Location: France

Who Was Studied: Adults receiving endotracheal mechanical ventilation for hypoxemic acute respiratory failure for no more than 48 hours, with a PaO_2:FiO_2 ratio greater than 300 mm Hg, new bilateral pulmonary infiltrates, and no evidence of left atrial hypertension (PCWP ≤ 18 mm Hg)

Who Was Excluded: Those with age < 18, known pregnancy, participation in another trial within 30 days, increased ICP, sickle cell disease, severe COPD requiring home oxygen or mechanical ventilation, weight exceeding 1kg/cm of height, severe burns, severe chronic liver disease, bone marrow transplant or chemotherapy-induced neutropenia, pneumothorax, expected duration of mechanical ventilation shorter than 48 hours, and decision to withhold life sustaining treatment.

How Many Patients: 767

Study Overview: Patients with ALI/ARDS were randomized to receive a PEEP strategy aimed at minimal alveolar distension versus increased alveolar recruitment (Figure 24.1).

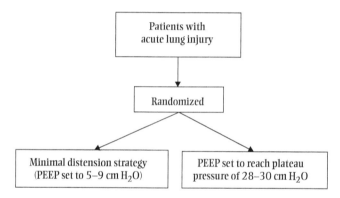

Figure 24.1 Summary of the study design.

Study Intervention: Both groups received goal tidal volumes of 6 mL per predicted body weight. Patients in the "minimal distension" (control) group received ventilation management targeted to achieve the lowest possible PEEP and plateau airway pressures without falling below oxygen goals (SpO_2 88%, PaO_2 55 mm Hg). External PEEP was set to maintain total PEEP between 5–9 mm H_2O.

Patients in the "increased recruitment" group had ventilation management targeted to increase PEEP to as high a level as possible without increasing maximal inspiratory airway plateau pressure above 28 to 30 cm H_2O. In this group, PEEP was titrated to plateau pressure regardless of oxygenation.

Follow-Up: 28 and 60 days

Endpoints: Primary outcome: 28 day mortality. Secondary outcomes: 60 day mortality, hospital censored mortality on day 60, number of ventilator-free days and organ failure–free days from day 1 to day 28, and the proportion of patients who experienced pneumothorax requiring chest tube drainage between day 1 and day 28.

RESULTS

- There was no difference in 28 day mortality between the minimal distension group and the increased recruitment group (31.2% vs. 27.8%; $p = 0.31$).
- There were significantly more ventilator-free days in the increased recruitment group (median 7 vs. 3 days) and organ failure–free days (median 6 vs. 2 days) compared with the minimal distension group.
- The increased recruitment group received less rescue therapy for refractory hypoxemia (34.6% vs. 18.7%; $p < 0.001$).
- There were no significant differences in incidence of pneumothorax between the minimal distension and increased recruitment groups (5.8% vs. 6.8%; $p = 0.57$).
- The increased recruitment group patients required significantly more fluid loading for hemodynamic support (amounting to approximately 400 mL over the first 72 hours) compared with the minimal distension group (Table 24.1).

Table 24.1. SUMMARY OF THE STUDY'S KEY FINDINGS

Outcome (in first 28 days)	Minimal Distension Group	Increased Recruitment Group	P Value
Mortality	31.2%	27.8%	0.31
Pneumothorax	5.8%	6.8%	0.57
Ventilator-free	3 (0–17)	7 (0–19)	0.04
Organ failure–free	2 (0–16)	6 (0–18)	0.04
Cardiovascular failure–free	21 (4–26)	23 (10–26)	0.09
Renal failure–free	27.5 (8–28)	28 (11–28)	0.23

Criticisms and Limitations:

- The study was unblinded, which could bias the results.
- Adjunctive interventions used in the case of severe hypoxemia (e.g., proning therapy and inhaled nitric oxide) were left to the discretion of the treating physician which could confound the results.
- In contrast to prior ARDS studies, relatively few of the patients in the ExPress trial presented with ARDS secondary to nonpulmonary causes, which raises questions regarding the generalizability of the findings.

Other Relevant Studies and Information:

- The ALVEOLI trial in 2004 examined higher versus lower PEEP, in conjunction with a low tidal volume and low plateau pressure strategy. A table linking FIO_2 and PEEP was created to guide up-titration or weaning of PEEP based on the required FIO_2. There was no significant difference in mortality, vent-free days, ICU free days, and organ failure–free days between groups.[2]
- The LOV randomized controlled trial examined the benefit of an "open-lung approach," to mechanical ventilation combining low tidal volume, lung recruitment maneuvers, and high positive-end–expiratory pressure in patients with ALI or ARDS. Similar to ExPress, the primary outcome showed no difference in mortality but supported previous findings of improved secondary outcomes of hypoxemia and rescue therapy utilization.[3]
- In 2013, Pintado et al. examined ventilatory management in the ARDS patient population with individualized PEEP settings aimed at obtaining the highest pulmonary compliance. The control arm followed low-volume ventilation and FIO_2 guided PEEP therapy. The compliance arm titrated PEEP once daily to achieve highest static compliance as measured during an inflation hold maneuver. The study outcomes identified an association with less organ dysfunction and a strong, nonsignificant trend toward lower mortality.[4]
- Secondary analysis of the LOVS and ExPress trial data identified oxygenation response to PEEP as a predictor of mortality in ARDS patients. Specifically, PEEP responsive patients had a lower risk of mortality.[5]
- Surviving sepsis campaign guidelines suggest using higher PEEP over lower PEEP in adult patients with sepsis-induced moderate to severe ARDS. This suggestion is based on the secondary analysis of the LOVS and ExPress trial data showing a survival benefit if PaO_2 / FiO_2 increased with higher PEEP.[6]

Summary and Implications: In mechanically ventilated patients with ALI/ARDS, there was no 28 or 60 day mortality benefit from an increased alveolar recruitment strategy (targeting PEEP to as high a level as possible without increasing maximal inspiratory airway plateau pressure above 28 to 30 cm H_2O) versus the standard minimal distension strategy (targeting PEEP of 5–9), However, there was a significant increase in ventilator free days and organ failure–free days, and no increased risk of pneumothorax with the utilization of the alveolar recruitment strategy.

CLINICAL CASE: PEEP IN ADULTS WITH ALI/ARDS

Case History:

A 63-year-old male admitted to the medical ICU with pneumonia and ARDS is treated with a mechanical ventilation PEEP strategy aimed at increased alveolar recruitment. A medical student asks you the benefits of this strategy. What is the best answer to this inquiry?

Suggested Answer:

The ExPress trial and others showed that a PEEP strategy aimed at increasing alveolar recruitment as opposed to minimal distension leads to improved oxygenation in severe ARDS, more ventilator-free days and fewer organ-failure days. A recent meta-analysis, which included data from the ExPress trial, revealed that higher levels of PEEP were associated with improved survival among patients with moderate to severe ARDS.[7] Current guidelines suggest using higher PEEP over lower PEEP in adult patients with sepsis-induced, moderate to severe ARDS.

References

1. Mercat A, Richard JC, Vielle B, et al. Positive end-expiratory pressure setting in adults with acute lung injury and acute respiratory distress syndrome: a randomized controlled trial. *JAMA*. 2008;299(6):646–655.
2. Brower RG, Lanken PN, Macintyre N, et al. Higher versus lower positive end-expiratory pressures in patients with the acute respiratory distress syndrome. *N Engl J Med*. 2004;351(4):327–336.
3. Meade MO, Cook DJ, Guyatt GH, et al. Ventilation strategy using low tidal volumes, recruitment maneuvers, and high positive end-expiratory pressure for acute lung injury and acute respiratory distress syndrome: a randomized controlled trial. *JAMA*. 2008;299(6):637–645.
4. Pintado MC, De Pablo R, Trascasa M, et al. Individualized PEEP setting in subjects with ARDS: a randomized controlled pilot study. *Respir Care*. 2013;58(9):1416–1423.
5. Goligher EC, Kavanagh BP, Rubenfeld GD, et al. Oxygenation response to positive end-expiratory pressure predicts mortality in acute respiratory distress syndrome. A secondary analysis of the LOVS and ExPress trials. *Am J Respir Crit Care Med*. 2014;190(1):70–76.
6. Rhodes A, Evans LE, Alhazzani W, et al. Surviving sepsis campaign: international guidelines for management of sepsis and septic shock: 2016. *Crit Care Med*. 2017;45(3):486–552.
7. Briel M, Meade M, Mercat A, et al. Higher vs lower positive end-expiratory pressure in patients with acute lung injury and acute respiratory distress syndrome: systematic review and meta-analysis. *JAMA*. 2010;303(9):865–873.

Efficacy and Safety of Corticosteroids for Persistent Acute Respiratory Distress Syndrome

SEAN LEVY AND EDNAN BAJWA

"Our results do not provide support for the routine use of methylprednisolone in patients with persistent ARDS and suggest that methylprednisolone therapy may be harmful when initiated more than two weeks after the onset of ARDS."

—STEINBERG ET AL.

Research Question: Are corticosteroids safe and effective in the treatment of persistent ARDS?[1]

Funding: The National Heart, Lung, and Blood Institute (NHLBI)

Year Study Began: 1997

Year Study Published: 2006

Study Location: 25 hospitals of the NHLBI ARDS Clinical Trials Network

Who Was Studied: Intubated patients receiving mechanical ventilation for clinically-defined ARDS for 7–28 days continuously with a PaO_2:FiO_2 ratio (adjusted for barometric pressure) less than 200 and persistent bilateral infiltrates on chest radiograph.

Who Was Excluded: Patients with serious infections (e.g., undrained abscess, intravascular infection, disseminated fungal infection, recent nosocomial pneumonia, or ongoing septic shock). All subjects were at least 13 years old and not pregnant. Those with burns requiring skin grafting, AIDS, recent cytotoxic therapy, or recent treatment with corticosteroids (greater than 300 mg prednisone, or its equivalent, cumulative dose within 21 days or greater than 15mg/day within 7 days prior to enrollment) were also excluded. Those subjects with an estimated 6-month mortality greater than 50%, severe chronic respiratory or liver disease, bone marrow or lung transplantation, known or suspected adrenal insufficiency, vasculitis or diffuse alveolar hemorrhage were excluded, as were those patients whose attending physician refused.

How Many Patients: 180 enrolled

Study Overview: See Figure 25.1 for an overview of the study design.

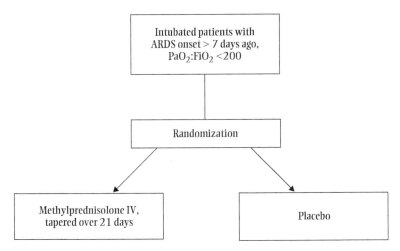

Figure 25.1 Summary of the study design.

Study Intervention: Those in the treatment arm received a single dose of methylprednisolone (2 mg/kg of predicted body weight), followed by a dose of 0.5 mg/kg predicted body weight every six hours for 14 days, followed by a dose of 0.5 mg/kg predicted body weight every twelve hours for 7 days, followed by further tapering over 2–4 days (see Figure 25.1). Subjects in both arms were weaned from the ventilator according to a pre-specified protocol. Particular attention was paid to the presence of new infections and hyperglycemia, and bronchoalveolar fluid and plasma were analyzed for inflammatory mediators.

Follow-Up: Subjects were followed until they died, were discharged home with unassisted breathing, or for 180 days, whichever came first.

Endpoints:

- *Primary outcome:* 60-day survival (defined as discharged home while breathing without assistance).
- *Secondary outcomes:* number of ventilator-free days, days without organ failure, and infectious complications during the first 28 days; changes in markers of inflammation and fibroproliferation at day 7. Additional information on outcomes at 180 days was also recorded.

RESULTS

- There was no difference between the steroid treatment (29.2%) and placebo (28.6%) groups in 60 day mortality ($p = 1.0$).
- There was no difference between the steroid treatment (31.5%) and placebo (31.9%) groups in 180-day mortality ($p = 1.0$)
- In those subjects with ARDS for greater than 14 days at the time of study entry, those in the steroid arm had higher 60-day and 180-day hospital mortality as compared with placebo ($p = 0.02$ and $p = 0.01$, respectively).
- After 28 days, there were more ventilator-free and shock-free days in the steroid group, along with improved respiratory-system compliance, oxygenation, and blood pressure, as defined as fewer days requiring vasopressor therapy.
- While overall rates of adverse events were similar, there was a higher rate of serious neuromyopathy in the steroid arm. Rates of nosocomial infection were similar between groups (Table 25.1).

Table 25.1. SUMMARY OF THE STUDY'S KEY FINDINGS

Outcome	Corticosteroid Group	Placebo Group	P-value
60-day hospital mortality	29.2%	28.6%	1.0
180-day hospital mortality	31.9%	31.5%	1.0
Ventilator-free days at 28 days	11.2 ± 9.4	6.8 ± 8.5	<0.001
60-day mortality (ARDS onset 7-13 days)	27%	36%	0.26
60-day mortality (ARDS onset > 14 days)	35%	8%	0.02

Criticisms and Limitations: The study was conducted over 7 years, during which a number of evidence-based advances in ARDS (including lung-protective ventilation)[2] and, more generally, in critical care, may have affected the outcomes. Additionally, in those patients who were extubated, steroids were tapered very rapidly in this study as compared with prior smaller studies that showed a benefit to steroids in persistent ARDS.[3] This may have negated any potential positive steroid effects.

Other Relevant Studies and Information:

- Corticosteroids have been shown to reduce inflammatory mediators in critical illnesses such as septic shock[4] and ARDS.[5] Abrupt cessation of steroids can produce a rebound in pro-inflammatory cytokines, providing an opportunity for continued inflammation and worse clinical outcomes.
- The role of corticosteroids in early (< 7 days onset) ARDS is not clear, with prior studies demonstrating mixed results.[6,7]
- A recent systematic review and meta-analysis concluded that current data do not support routine use of corticosteroids in ARDS.

Summary and Implications: In patients with ARDS lasting > 7 days, corticosteroids did not improve overall mortality as compared with placebo. Steroids did improve secondary outcomes, such as ventilator-free and shock-free days, and were associated with lower rates of septic shock and pneumonia.

CLINICAL CASE: TO SALVAGE OR NOT TO SALVAGE

Case History:
A sixty-four-year-old man with no known prior lung disease presents with septic shock and ARDS that are attributed to pneumonia. After eight days of continuous mechanical ventilation, his PaO_2:FiO_2 ratio remains less than 150 and his respiratory system compliance (as measured by the ventilator) is poor. He continues to require vasopressors for septic shock. Given his lack of improvement, the decision to administer corticosteroids as a "salvage" intervention is considered.

Suggested Answer:
The patient's clinical status is similar to that of the subjects in the trial examining the safety and efficacy of corticosteroids in persistent ARDS.[1] As with all patients with ARDS, he should be treated with lung-protective ventilation with limited tidal volumes and plateau pressures, in order to reduce the likelihood of ventilator-induced lung injury (VILI). He should not be administered corticosteroids solely for the treatment of ARDS. Should he require corticosteroids for an alternative indication, such as refractory shock, however, these steroids should be tapered slowly, even in the event of liberation from mechanical liberation, in order to reduce the likelihood of a rebound of inflammatory mediators potentially contributing to worsened gas exchange.

References

1. Steinberg KP, Hudson LD, Goodman RB, et al. Efficacy and safety of corticosteroids for persistent acute respiratory distress syndrome. *N Engl J Med.* 2006; 354: 1671–84.
2. The Acute Respiratory Distress Syndrome Network. Ventilation with lower tidal volumes as compared with traditional tidal volumes for acute lung injury and the acute respiratory distress syndrome. *N Engl J Med.* 2000; 342: 1301–8.
3. Meduri GU, Headley AS, Golden E, et al. Effect of prolonged methylprednisolone therapy in unresolving acute respiratory distress syndrome. *JAMA.* 1998; 280: 159–65.
4. Keh D, Boehnke T, Weber-Cartens S, et al. Immunologic and hemodynamic effects of "low-dose" hydrocortisone in septic shock. *Am J Respir Crit Care Med.* 2003; 167: 512–20.
5. Seam N, Meduri GU, Wang H, et al. Effects of methylprednisolone infusion on markers of inflammation, coagulation, and angiogenesis in early acute respiratory distress syndrome. *Crit Care Med.* 2012; 40: 495–501.
6. Bernard GR, Luce JM, Sprung CL, et al. High-dose corticosteroids in patients with the acute respiratory distress syndrome. *N Engl J Med.* 1987; 317: 1565–70.
7. Meduri GU, Golden E, Freire AX, et al. Methylprednisolone infusion in early severe ARDS. *Chest.* 2007; 131: 954–63.

26

Effect of Early versus Late Tracheostomy Placement on Survival in Patients Receiving Mechanical Ventilation

The TracMan Trial

J. MICHAEL GUTHRIE AND VADIM GUDZENKO

> "Among mechanically ventilated critically ill patients in adult, general critical care units in the United Kingdom, early tracheostomy (within the first 4 days after admission) was not associated with an improvement in 30-day mortality or other important secondary outcomes."
> —THE TRACMAN COLLABORATORS

Research Question: Does early versus late tracheostomy lower mortality in mechanically ventilated critically ill patients?[1]

Funding: The Intensive Care Society and the Medical Research Council, both in the United Kingdom

Year Study Began: 2004

Year Study Published: 2013

Study Location: 70 adult general ICUs and 2 cardiothoracic ICUs in 13 university and 39 non-university hospitals in the United Kingdom

Who Was Studied: Mechanically ventilated patients identified by the treating clinician in the first 4 days after admission as likely to need at least 7 more days of mechanical ventilation.

Who Was Excluded: Patients who required immediate life-saving tracheostomy, patients for whom tracheostomy was contraindicated due anatomical or other reasons, and patients with respiratory failure caused by chronic neurologic disease.

How Many Patients: 1032 patients approached for participation; 909 patients were randomized

Study Overview: This study examined mortality among patients randomized to receive early (first 4 days) versus late (after 10 days) tracheostomy (see Figure 26.1).

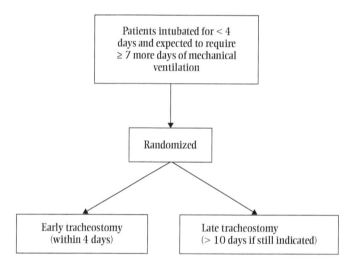

Figure 26.1 Summary of the study design.

Study Intervention: Patients randomized to the early tracheostomy group received a tracheostomy within four days of intensive care unit admission. Patients randomized to the late tracheostomy group received a tracheostomy on day 10 or later, and only if the treating clinician deemed tracheostomy still necessary. Tracheostomies could be either surgical or percutaneous.

Follow-Up: 2 years

End Points: The Primary Outcome was all cause mortality 30 days after randomization. Secondary outcomes were mortality at ICU discharge, hospital discharge, 1 year and 2 years, length of stay in the ICU and hospital, number of days in ICU during which IV sedatives were administered from admission to 30 days, number of antimicrobial free days in ICU from admission to 30 days (used as a surrogate marker for hospital acquired infections).

RESULTS

- 909 patients randomized, 455 to early tracheostomy and 455 to late tracheostomy.
- 899 patients were included for final analysis. 451 patients in early group and 448 patients in late group. The 10 missing patients were not included due to duplicate randomization and patient withdrawal from the study.
- Medical admission comprised 79.2% of the patients with 20.8% being surgical.
- In the early tracheostomy group 385 patients (84.6%) received tracheostomy within 4 days of admission.
- For the 66 early tracheostomy group patients who did not receive tracheostomy within 4 days:
  - 4 died before tracheostomy.
  - 11 recovered and did not need tracheostomy.
  - 16 remained too unstable to receive tracheostomy.
  - 19 received tracheostomy after 4 days because they were too unstable in the first 4 days.
  - 6 received tracheostomy after day 4 because they had unavailable facilities or operators.
  - 4 initially improved then went on to need tracheostomy after 4 days.
  - 2 received tracheostomy after 4 days due to investigator error.
  - 4 received late tracheostomy due to unknown reasons.
- In the late tracheostomy group 55% of the patients never had a tracheostomy performed:
  - 36.8% patients in the late group never received a tracheostomy because they improved and no longer required mechanical ventilation at day 10.
  - Among the remaining late tracheostomy patients who did not receive the procedure, 54 died, 11 remained too unstable, 2 had treatment withdrawn, and 10 had no recorded reason.
- The rate of tracheostomy related complications was similar between groups; 6.3% in the early group and 7.8% late group.
- 30-day mortality, the primary outcome, was not different between the early and late tracheostomy groups at 30.8% and 31.5%, respectively.
- Mortality at ICU discharge, hospital discharge, 1 year and 2 years was not different between the early and late tracheostomy groups.

- ICU length of stay was not different between early and late tracheostomy groups.
- Antibiotic use was similar in the two groups.
- Among survivors, patients in the late group had more days receiving sedatives (Table 26.1).

Table 26.1. SUMMARY OF TRACMAN'S KEY FINDINGS

Outcome	Early Tracheostomy (n = 451)	Late Tracheostomy (n = 448)	P Value
30 Day Mortality	30.8%	31.5%	0.89
2 Year Mortality	51%	53.4%	0.42
Complication Rate	5.5%	7.8%	NS

Criticisms and Limitations:

- This study did not succeed in enrolling its intended number of patients and was underpowered.
- The study accrued patients at a rate of less than 2 patients per site per year, leaving significant potential for inconsistent recruitment and variance in clinical practice.
- The decision to enroll patients in the study was driven by clinician assessment instead of a decision tool to predict which patients would need prolonged mechanical ventilation.
- This study did not include neuro-critical care patients, a cohort that frequently requires tracheostomy.
- The study was not designed or powered to assess other potential complications of late tracheostomy such as laryngotracheal stenosis, In addition voice, swallowing, and airway rehabilitation might benefit by earlier tracheostomy.
- Patient comfort is another potential benefit with early tracheostomy. The study did not report the use of pain medications.
- The use of day 10 for late tracheostomy is entirely arbitrary. The study results do not provide insight into the ideal timing of tracheostomy.

Other Relevant Studies and Information:

- Initial small trials suggested a mortality benefit to early tracheostomy but later larger and better-conducted trials have tended to show no benefit.[2, 3]
- Terragani randomized 419 patients to early (after 6–8 days of intubation) versus late (after 13–15 days of intubation) tracheostomy with a primary outcome of rate of ventilator associated pneumonia, and found no difference between groups. As with the TracMan

trial a significant number of patients recovered and did not require tracheostomy.[4]

- A randomized controlled trial of early versus late tracheostomy in 216 cardiac surgical patients found no difference in number of ventilator free days, ventilator associated infection or survival.[5] However, early tracheotomy was associated with less sedation, less delirium, fewer unscheduled extubations, better comfort, and earlier resumption of oral nutrition.
- A metanalysis of 14 RCTs of early versus late tracheostomy failed to demonstrate any difference between groups in short-term mortality, ventilator-free days, ventilator associated PNA, or long-term mortality.[6]
- Recent guidelines suggest that the optimal timing of tracheostomy be determined on an individual patient basis. There is insufficient or conflicting evidence to make a general recommendation of early versus late tracheostomy.[7]

Summary and Implications: For most patients with prolonged respiratory failure, early tracheostomy does not improve mortality, nor does it improve patient important outcomes such as ICU or hospital length of stay. Additionally, clinicians' ability to predict which ICU patients will require prolonged mechanical ventilation is severely limited, as many patients predicted to need prolonged mechanical ventilatory support will actually recover. A strategy of early tracheostomy would result in a significant number of patients receiving unnecessary tracheostomies and a small but real number suffering complications without improving mortality. Thus in most mechanically ventilated ICU patients, tracheostomy should be delayed until at least 10 days.

CLINICAL CASE: EFFECT OF EARLY VERSUS LATE TRACHEOSTOMY PLACEMENT ON SURVIVAL IN PATIENTS RECEIVING MECHANICAL VENTILATION

Case History:
A 69-year-old male is admitted to the ICU with community acquired pneumonia and develops acute respiratory distress syndrome (ARDS). He is intubated in the emergency department and is still requiring mechanical ventilation on hospital day 2. Based on the results of TracMan should this patient receive early tracheostomy?

Suggested Answer:
Given that this patient developed ARDS from pneumonia he may well require prolonged mechanical ventilation. However, the results of this study

suggest that clinicians frequently predict that patients will require prolonged mechanical ventilation only to have them recover before 10 days. Additionally, the study failed to demonstrate a mortality benefit attributable to early tracheostomy. Therefore tracheostomy should be delayed for at least 10 days in this patient.

References

1. Young D, Harrison DA, Cuthbertson BH, Rowan K; TracMan Collaborators. Effect of early vs late tracheostomy placement on survival in patients receiving mechanical ventilation: the TracMan randomized trial. *JAMA*. 2013;309(20):2121–2129.
2. Arabi Y, Haddad S, Shirawi N, Al SA. Early tracheostomy in intensive care trauma patients improves resource utilization: a cohort study and literature review. *Crit Care*. 2004;8(5):R347–352.
3. Griffiths J, Barber VS, Morgan L, Young JD. Systematic review and meta-analysis of studies of the timing of tracheostomy in adult patients undergoing artificial ventilation. *BMJ*. 2005;330(7502):1243.
4. Terragni PP, Antonelli M, Fumagalli R, et al. Early vs late tracheotomy for prevention of pneumonia in mechanically ventilated adult ICU patients: a randomized controlled trial. *JAMA*. 2010;303(15):1483–1489.
5. Trouillet JL, Luyt CE, Guiguet M, et al. Early percutaneous tracheotomy versus prolonged intubation of mechanically ventilated patients after cardiac surgery: a randomized trial. *Ann Intern Med*. 2011;154:373–383.
6. Szakmany T, Russell P, Wilkes AR, Hall JE. Effect of early tracheostomy on resource utilization and clinical outcomes in critically ill patients: meta-analysis of randomized controlled trials. *Br J Anaesth*. 2015;114(3):396–405.
7. Madsen KR, Guldager H, Rewers M, Weber SO, et al. Danish guidelines 2015 for percutaneous dilatational tracheostomy in the intensive care unit. *Dan Med J*. 2015;62(3). pii: B5042.

27

Using Esophageal Pressures to Improve Oxygenation and Compliance in Acute Lung Injury

CONNIE WANG AND EDWARD BITTNER

"Oxygenation and respiratory-system compliance improved in the esophageal-pressure-guided group as compared with the control group... these improvements in lung function were associated with a trend toward improved 28-day survival."

—TALMOR D, ET AL.

Research Question: Can the use of pleural pressure measurements obtained by esophageal manometry be used to find a PEEP value that can maintain oxygenation while preventing lung injury in patients with acute respiratory distress syndrome (ARDS)?[1]

Sponsor: Supported in part by a grant from the National Heart, Lung, and Blood Institute

Year Study Began: 2004

Year Study Published: 2008

Study Location: Medical and surgical intensive care units of Beth Israel Deaconess Medical Center in Boston.

Who Was Studied: Patients who had ALI or ARDS that fit the American-European Consensus Conference definition (See Box 27.1).

Box 27.1. THE AMERICAN-EUROPEAN CONSENSUS DEFINITION FOR ALI/ARDS

Definition of Acute Lung Injury (ALI) and Acute Respiratory Distress Syndrome (ARDS)

1. Acute injury of a suggestive etiology
2. Diffuse bilateral infiltrates on chest radiograph
3. Severe hypoxemia: PaO_2/FiO_2 < 300 mm Hg for ALI and < 200 mm Hg for ARDS
4. Absence of cardiac failure: wedge pressure < 18 mm Hg (no left atrial hypertension).[2]

Who Was Excluded: Patients were excluded if they had recent trauma or pathology of the esophagus, significant bronchopleural fistula, and solid-organ transplantation.

How Many Patients: 61

Study Overview: See Figure 27.1 for a summary of the study's design.

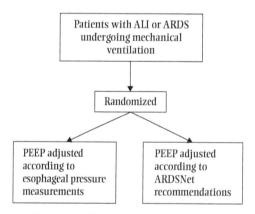

Figure 27.1 Summary of the study design.

Study Intervention: All subjects had an esophageal balloon catheter inserted to estimate pleural pressure from measured esophageal pressure. In the esophageal-pressure guided group the tidal volume was set to 6 mL per kilogram of predicted body weight and positive end-expiratory pressure (PEEP) levels were set to achieve a transpulmonary pressure (difference between the airway pressure and the esophageal pressure) of 0 to 10 cm of water at end expiration according to a sliding scale (based on partial pressure of arterial oxygen $[PaO_2]$ and fraction of inspired oxygen $[FiO_2]$). Patients in the control group were managed according to the ARDSNet Study protocol utilizing low tidal volumes of 6 mL per kilogram of predicted weight and PEEP based on patient's PaO_2 and FiO_2.[3] In both arms, the objectives of mechanical ventilation included a PaO_2 between 55 and 120 mm Hg or oxygen saturation between 88% and 98% by pulse oximetry, partial pressure of arterial carbon dioxide $(PaCO_2)$ from 40 to 60 mm Hg and an arterial pH ranging between 7.30 and 7.45.

Follow-Up: Measurements were performed at 5 minutes from initiation of the intervention or controlled ventilation and follow-up measurements were repeated at 24, 48, and 72 hours. Additional measurements were performed if changes were made to ventilator settings because of changes in the patient's clinical condition.

Endpoints: Primary endpoint: arterial oxygenation measured by the ratio of $PaO_2{:}FiO_2$ at 72 hours. Secondary endpoints: measures of respiratory system compliance and physiological dead space, number of ventilator-free days at 28 days, length of stay in the ICU, death within 28 days and 180 days after treatment.

RESULTS

- The PaO_2/FiO_2 ratio at 72 hours was 88 mm Hg higher in the esophageal-pressure– guided group than in the control group. This effect was persistent at 24, 48, and 72 hours.
- Respiratory-system compliance was also significantly better at 24, 48, and 72 hours in the esophageal pressure–guided group compared with the control group.

After adjustment for baseline APACHE II scores the esophageal-pressure protocol was associated with a significant reduction in 28-day mortality as compared with treatment in the control group (Table 27.1).

Table 27.1. SUMMARY OF THE STUDY'S KEY FINDINGS

Measurement	Baseline Esophageal-Pressure-Guided	Conventional Treatment	P Value	72 Hours Esophageal-Pressure-Guided	Conventional Treatment	P Value
$PaO_2{:}FiO_2$	147+/−56	145+/−57	0.89	280+/−126	191+/−71	0.002
Respiratory-system compliance	36+/−12	36+/−10	0.98	45+/−14	35+/−9	0.005
PEEP (cm of water)	13+/−5	13+/−3	0.73	17+/−6	10+/−4	< 0.001
Tidal volume (mL per kg of predicated body weight)	7.3+/−1.3	7.9+/−1.4	0.12	7.1+/−1.3	6.8+/−1	0.31
Plateau pressure (cm of water)	29+/−7	29+/−5	0.79	28+/−7	25+/−6	0.07
Transpulmonary end-expiratory pressure (cm of water)	−2.8+/5.0	-1.9+/−4.7	0.49	0.1+/−2.6	−2.0+/−4.7	0.06

Plus-minus values are means +/-SD. FiO$_2$ denotes fraction of inspired oxygen, PaO$_2$ the partial pressure of arterial oxygen, PEEP positive end-expiratory pressure applied by the ventilator, and PEEP total airway pressure measured during end-expiratory occlusion (Table 27.2).

Table 27.2. CLINICAL OUTCOMES

Outcome	Esophageal-Pressure-Guided (N = 30)	Conventional Treatment (N = 31)	P Value
28-Day mortality—no. (%)	5 (17)	12 (39)	0.06
180-Day mortality—no. (%)	8 (27)	14 (45)	0.13
Length of ICU stay—days	15.5	13	0.16
Number of ICU-free days at 28 days	5	4	0.96
Number of ventilator-free days at 28 days	11.5	7	0.5
Number of days of ventilation among survivors	12	16	0.71

Criticisms and Limitations:

- Limitations of this study include a single center with a small sample size. A larger trial powered to detect changes in appropriate clinical end points is needed for definitive conclusions.
- The primary end point was oxygenation, which has previously been shown to improve by applied PEEP.[4] In addition, prior studies have demonstrated improvement in oxygenation at the cost of higher airway pressures to have either no effect or an increased mortality.[3,5,6] Hence, the favorable outcomes observed in this study need to be validated with larger trials assessing hard clinical endpoints.
- An extrapulmonary cause of the ARDS was present in a high proportion of patients in the study (39%). The increase in the intra-abdominal pressure, which has been shown to be greater in extrapulmonary ARDS, could explain the benefit observed in the study. It is possible that populations of patients with pulmonary ARDS, which does not involve any major changes in the compliance of the chest wall, will not benefit from measurement of esophageal pressure to set PEEP.

Other Relevant Studies and Information:

- Even though several animal models which have shown that increasing PEEP in acute lung injury can be protective against lung injury in reducing end-expiratory lung volume or pressure,[7–9] several large randomized control trials in human adults have not shown beneficial effects from low PEEP compared to higher values of PEEP.[5, 6, 10]

- A meta-analysis evaluating 3 trials with 2299 patients showed that higher values of PEEP compared to lower values in patients with ALI or ARDS were not associated with an improvement in hospital mortality. However, higher PEEP values were seen to be associated with an improved survival for among the subgroup of patients with ARDS.[11] The Esophageal Pressure-Guided Ventilation 2 (EPVent2) trial is a multicenter, prospective, randomized, phase II clinical trial currently enrolling patients to test the hypothesis that the use of a transpulmonary pressure -guided ventilation strategy will lead to improvement in composite outcomes of mortality and time off the ventilator at 28 days as compared with a high-PEEP control.[12]

Summary and Implications: This study suggests that a ventilation strategy using esophageal manometry to optimize transpulmonary pressure is feasible and may be superior to ventilator adjustments based on the ARDS Network protocol, which is the current standard of care. Further validation in larger studies assessing hard clinical endpoints is required before this can be considered the standard of care, however.

CLINICAL CASE: USING ESOPHAGEAL MANOMETRY TO GUIDE MECHANICAL VENTILATION

Case History:
A 38-year-old man is admitted to the ICU with necrotizing pancreatitis. His course is complicated by abdominal compartment syndrome which required urgent decompression. Chest x-ray shows acute onset bilateral infiltrates and, despite recruitment maneuvers and use of high PEEP, the patient's gas exchange remains poor with a PaO_2/FiO_2 ratio of 175. Based on the results of this study, what would you advise a colleague who inquires about the utility of placing an esophageal balloon to help guide management?

Suggested Answer:
High abdominal pressures in this case of increased intra-abdominal pressure might alter chest wall mechanics. Based on this study, the use of esophageal pressure measurements could better guide optimal PEEP with improvement in oxygenation and lung compliance, as well as 28 day survival. However, several considerations need to be taken into account before using esophageal

balloon manometry to guide optimal PEEP levels. Catheter insertion has its own associated risks and can often be difficult to place. The correct position is in the lower one-third of the esophagus behind the heart.[1] A patient's body position can also affect measurements and adequate compensation for positional artifact should be accounted for.[12, 13] Patients with lung injury may also not have equal transpulmonary pressures due to varying degrees of consolidation throughout the different regions of the lung. Once these factors are taken into consideration, based on the results of this clinical study, insertion of esophageal balloon could potentially help improve this patient's oxygenation.

References

1. Talmor D, Sarge T, Malhotra A, O'Donnell CR, Ritz R, Lisbon A, Novack V, Loring SH. Mechanical ventilation guided by esophageal pressure in acute lung injury. *N Engl J Med*. 2008;359(20):2095–2104.
2. Bernard GR, Artigas A, Brigham KL, et al. The American-European Consensus Conference on ARDS: definitions, mechanisms, relevant outcomes, and clinical trial coordination. *Am J Respir Crit Care Med*. 1994;149:818–824.
3. The Acute Respiratory Distress Syndrome Network. Ventilation with lower tidal volumes as compared with traditional tidal volumes for acute lung injury and the acute respiratory distress syndrome. *N Engl J Med*. 2000;342:1301–1308.
4. Villar J, Perez-Mendez L, Lopez J, et al. An early PEEP/FIO$_2$ trial identifies different degrees of lung injury in patients with acute respiratory distress syndrome. *Am J Respir Crit Care Med*. 2007;176:795–804.
5. Meade MO, Cook DJ, Guyatt GH, et al. Ventilation strategy using low tidal volumes, recruitment maneuvers, and high positive end-expiratory pressure for acute lung injury and acute respiratory distress syndrome: a randomized controlled trial. *JAMA*. 2008;299:637–645.
6. Mercat A, Richard JC, Vielle B, et al. Positive end-expiratory pressure setting in adults with acute lung injury and acute respiratory distress syndrome: a randomized controlled trial. *JAMA*. 2008;299:646–655.
7. Chiumello D, Pristine G, Slutsky AS. Mechanical ventilation affects local and systemic cytokines in an animal model of acute respiratory distress syndrome. *Am J Respir Crit Care Med*. 1999;160:109–116.
8. Faridy EE, Permutt S, Riley RL. Effect of ventilation on surface forces in excised dogs' lungs. *J Appl Physiol*. 1966;21:1453–1462.
9. Muscedere JG, Mullen JB, Gan K, Slutsky AS. Tidal ventilation at low airway pressures can augment lung injury. *Am J Respir Crit Care Med*. 1994;149:1327–1334.
10. Brower RG, Lanken PN, MacIntyre N, et al. Higher versus lower positive end-expiratory pressures in patients with the acute respiratory distress syndrome. *N Engl J Med*. 2004; 351:327–336.
11. Briel M, Meade M, Mercat A, et al. Higher vs lower positive end-expiratory pressure in patients with acute lung injury and acute respiratory distress syndrome: systematic review and metaanalysis. *JAMA*. 2010; 303:865–873.

12. Fish E, Novack V, Banner-Goodspeed VM, et al. The Esophageal Pressure-Guided Ventilation 2 (EPVent2) trial protocol: a multicentre, randomised clinical trial of mechanical ventilation guided by transpulmonary pressure. *BMJ Open*. 2014;4(9):e006356.
13. Washko GR, O'Donnell CR, Loring SH. Volume-related and volume-independent effects of posture on esophageal and transpulmonary pressures in healthy subjects. *J Appl Physiol*. (1985). 2006;100(3):753–758.

A Comparison of Four Methods of Weaning Patients from Mechanical Ventilation

SHERI BERG AND ARCHIT SHARMA

"A once-daily trial of spontaneous breathing led to extubation about three times more quickly than intermittent mandatory ventilation and about twice as quickly as pressure-support ventilation. Multiple daily trials of spontaneous breathing were equally successful."

—ESTEBAN ET AL.

Research Question: What is the best method for weaning mechanical ventilation in patients with an initial unsuccessful spontaneous breathing trial?[1]

Funding: Supported in part by a grant from the Veterans Affairs Research Service

Year Study Began: 1992

Year Study Published: 1995

Study Location: 14 medical-surgical intensive care units of 14 teaching hospitals in Spain.

Who Was Studied: Patients who received mechanical ventilation for more than 24 hours, due to acute respiratory failure and with "improvement in or resolution of the underlying cause of acute respiratory failure and a ratio of artieral oxygen to inspired oxygen $(PaO_2/FiO_2) > 200$ with a positive end-expiratory pressure

(PEEP) ≤5 cm H$_2$O, a temperature < 38°C; a hemoglobin level > 10 g/dl and no need for vasoactive and sedative agents.

Who Was Excluded: Patients with a tracheostomy, a temperature ≥ 38°C; a hemoglobin level ≤ 10 g/dl, or those with an ongoing need for vasoactive and sedative agents.

How Many Patients: 130

Study Overview: Patients who failed a 2 hour spontaneous breathing trial via a t-tube were designated as "difficult to wean" and randomly assigned to one of the following weaning strategies:

- Intermittent Mandatory Ventilation (IMV)—initial rate of 10 breaths per minute (bpm), then decreased at least twice a day as tolerated.
- Pressure Support Ventilation (PSV)—initially set at 18 cm H$_2$O then reduced by 2 to 4 cm H$_2$O at least twice a day.
- A once a day Spontaneous Breathing Trial (SBT) with mechanical ventilation between trials.
- Intermittent SBT trials at least twice daily with mechanical ventilation between trials.

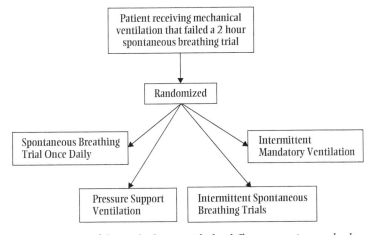

Figure 28.1 Summary of the study design with the different weaning methods.

Patients were extubated if they tolerated a trial for 2 hours (Figure 28.1).

Follow-Up: For all four methods, weaning was deemed successful if extubation was achieved within the 14-day time period and reintubation was not required within 48 hours of extubation.

Endpoints: Time to successful extubation

RESULTS

- Four factors predicted the time required for successful weaning: age, the duration of mechanical ventilation before weaning was begun, the time to the failure of the first SBT and weaning technique.
- The median duration of weaning was 5 (interquartile range, IQR, 3–11) days for intermittent mandatory ventilation, 4 (IQR 2–12) for pressure-support ventilation, 3 (2 and 6) days for intermittent (multiple) trials of spontaneous breathing, and 3 (1–6) days for a once-daily trial of spontaneous breathing.
- The rate of successful weaning was higher with a once-daily trial of spontaneous breathing than with intermittent mandatory ventilation or pressure-support ventilation.
- There was no significant difference in the rate of successful weaning between once-daily trials and multiple trials of spontaneous breathing (Table 28.1).

Table 28.1. RESULTS OF SUCCESSFUL WEANING WITH DIFFERENT TECHNIQUES

Weaning technique	Relative rate of successful weaning and (95% confidence interval)	p-value
Once daily SBT vs. IMV	2.83 (1.36–5.89)	0.006
Once-daily SBT vs. PSV	2.05 (1.04–4.04)	0.04
Once-daily SBT vs. intermittent SBT	1.24 (0.64–2.41)	0.54

Criticism and Limitations: Despite the use of randomization, the patients in the group assigned to intermittent mandatory ventilation had received ventilation for a shorter time than the patients in the other groups. This resulted in a bias in their favor, since weaning is accomplished more rapidly in patients receiving short-term support.

- Because the trial was small, a few outliers (e.g., patients who were extremely difficult to wean because of their underlying pulmonary disease) in any particular group could affect outcomes. The studies' results apply only to the specific weaning protocol used in the study. It is possible that the other methods may be better for some subgroups of patients, or that differences in the details of the weaning protocols would have yielded different results.

- How some combination of intermittent mandatory ventilation and pressure-support ventilation might compare with other methods of weaning is unknown.

Other Relevant Studies and Information:

- Evidence suggests that standardized weaning protocols reduce the duration of mechanical ventilation, weaning duration, and ICU length of stay compared with nonprotocolized weaning especially among patients in medical, surgical, and mixed ICUs, but not in neurosurgical ICUs.[2]
- A recent metaanalysis comparing the duration of weaning from mechanical ventilation for critically ill ventilated patients found that automated closed loop systems may result in reduced duration of weaning, ventilation, and ICU stay when compared with non-automated strategies.[3]
- Some observational studies suggest that reintubation rates are significantly higher when SBTs are performed with the use of CPAP compared with T-tube tests or low pressure support without PEEP. However, randomized trials do not provide evidence of a higher reintubation risk between those methods.[4]
- Strong evidence suggests that SBTs should be at least 30 min but not longer than 120 min.[5,6] Well-defined criteria for terminating an SBT do not exist, and currently, trials are terminated on the basis of clinical judgment.
- Current guidelines recommend spontaneous breathing trials regularly to evaluate the ability to discontinue mechanical ventilation.[7,8]

Summary and Implications: Among carefully selected patients who were difficult to wean from the ventilator, a once-daily trial of spontaneous breathing led to extubation about three times more quickly than intermittent mandatory ventilation and about twice as quickly as pressure-support ventilation. There was no significant difference in the rate of success between a once-daily trial and multiple daily trials of spontaneous breathing or between intermittent mandatory ventilation and pressure-support ventilation.

CLINICAL CASE: MODE OF WEANING FROM MECHANICAL VENTILATION

Case History:
A 76-year-old man is admitted to the ICU respiratory failure from community acquired pneumonia and requires mechanical ventilation for 5 days. He is

now awake, following commands, hemodynamically stable, and has an oxygen saturation of 98% with an FiO_2 of 30% on PEEP of 5 cm H_2O. A spontaneous breathing trial is attempted but he fails within 30 minutes due to tachypnea with low tidal volumes and he is placed back on mechanical ventilation. Based on the results of the trial, what mode of mechanical ventilation should be used in weaning this patient?

Suggested Answer:

For patients that fail an initial trial of spontaneous breathing, this study showed that spontaneous breathing trials are superior for weaning patients from mechanical ventilation compared with intermittent mandatory ventilation or pressure support ventilation. Spontaneous breathing trials have a higher probability of success and result in a shorter duration of mechanical ventilation. Once-daily spontaneous breathing trials appear to be equivalent to intermittent breathing trials more than once a day. The patient in this vignette is similar to those included in the trial and therefore should be weaned using a once-daily spontaneous breathing trial.

References

1. Esteban A, Frutos F, Tobin MJ, et al. A comparison of four methods of weaning patients from mechanical ventilation. Spanish Lung Failure Collaborative Group. *N Engl J Med.* 1995;332(6):345–350.
2. Blackwood B, Burns KE, Cardwell CR, O'Halloran P. Protocolized versus non-protocolized weaning for reducing the duration of mechanical ventilation in critically ill adult patients. *Cochrane Database Syst Rev.* 2014;6(11):CD006904.
3. Rose L, Schultz MJ, Cardwell CR, Jouvet P, McAuley DF, Blackwood B. Automated versus non-automated weaning for reducing the duration of mechanical ventilation for critically ill adults and children. *Cochrane Database Syst Rev.* 2014;10(6):CD009235.
4. Peñuelas Ó, Thille AW, Esteban A. Discontinuation of ventilatory support: new solutions to old dilemmas. *Curr Opin Crit Care.* 2015;21(1):74–81.
5. Ely EW, Baker AM, Dunagan DP, et al. Effect on the duration of mechanical ventilation of identifying patients capable of breathing spontaneously. *N Engl J Med.* 1996;335:1864–1869.
6. Vallverdu´ I, Calaf N, Subirana M, et al. Clinical characteristics, respiratory functional parameters, and outcome of a two-hour T-piece trial in patients weaning from mechanical ventilation. *Am J Respir Crit Care Med.* 1998; 158:1855–1862.
7. Society for Healthcare Epidemiology of America (SHEA). Strategies to prevent ventilator-associated pneumonia in acute care hospitals: 2014 update. *Infect Control Hosp Epidemiol.* 2014;35(8):915–936.
8. Surviving sepsis campaign: international guidelines for management of sepsis and septic shock: 2016. *Intensive Care Med.* 2017;43(3):304–377.

29

Noninvasive Ventilation for Acute COPD Exacerbations

ROBERT LOFLIN AND DAVID KAUFMAN

"In selected patients with acute exacerbations of chronic obstructive pulmonary disease, noninvasive ventilation can reduce the need for endotracheal intubation, the length of hospital stay, and the in-hospital mortality rate."

—BROCHARD ET AL.

Research Question: In patients with acute exacerbations of chronic obstructive pulmonary disease (COPD), does noninvasive positive pressure ventilation (NPPV) delivered via facemask reduce the need for endotracheal intubation and mechanical ventilation, hospital length of stay, and mortality?[1]

Funding: Not described

Year Study Began: 1990

Year Study Published: 1995

Study Location: 5 hospitals in France (3), Italy (1), and Spain (1)

Who Was Studied: Adult patients with acute COPD exacerbations

Who Was Excluded: Patients with a tracheotomy or endotracheal intubation performed prior to admission; the administration of sedative drugs within the previous 12 hours; a central nervous system disorder unrelated to hypercapnic encephalopathy or hypoxemia; cardiac arrest; cardiogenic pulmonary edema; kyphoscoliosis or a neuromuscular disorder as the cause of chronic respiratory failure; upper airway obstruction or asthma; a clear cause of decompensation requiring specific treatment (e.g., peritonitis, septic shock, acute myocardial infarction, pulmonary thromboembolism, pneumothorax, hemoptysis, severe pneumonia, or recent surgery or trauma); a facial deformity; or patients who refused to undergo endotracheal intubation.

How Many Patients: 85

Study Overview: Multicenter, prospective, randomized trial to compare the efficacy of NPPV, delivered through a face mask, with standard medical treatment, in patients admitted with acute exacerbations of chronic obstructive pulmonary disease (Figure 29.1).

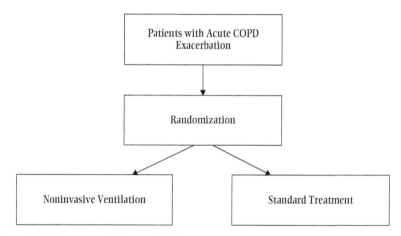

Figure 29.1 Summary of the study design.

Study Intervention: Patients in the NPPV group received flow-triggered, pressure-limited, flow-cycled pressure support ventilation delivered via a novel face-mask developed for use in the study. Initial settings included 20 cm H_2O inspiratory pressure support above atmospheric pressure for expiratory support. Supplemental oxygen was titrated to achieve an arterial oxygen saturation above 90%. Treatment was provided for at least 6 hours each day with the duration extended depending upon patient tolerance and clinical assessment. Patients in the standard treatment group received supplemental oxygen via nasal prongs with a maximal flow rate of 5 L/min titrated to maintain arterial oxygen saturation above 90%.

Follow-Up: All patients had arterial blood gas measurements and clinical scoring at 1, 3, and 12 hours after start of treatment. Pulmonary function testing was performed prior to discharge if possible or within 3 months.

Endpoints: The primary outcome was the need for endotracheal intubation. Secondary outcomes included the duration of ventilator assistance, length of stay, in-hospital mortality, and complications such as pneumonia, barotrauma, gastrointestinal hemorrhage, renal insufficiency, neurologic events, and pulmonary embolism.

RESULTS

- Medical treatment provided for acute COPD exacerbation was similar in both groups, including use of antibiotics, corticosteroids, and bronchodilators
- In the NPPV group, 26% of patients required endotracheal intubation compared to 74% of patients in the standard treatment group; $P < 0.001$.
- Patients treated with NPPV had improvement in encephalopathy score, respiratory rate, PaO_2, and pH after 1 hour of treatment
- Complications, including pneumonia and sepsis, were significantly higher in the standard group (48%) compared to the NPPV group (16%); $P = 0.001$
- Length of hospital stay was higher in the standard group (35 +/− 33 days) compared to the NPPV group (23 +/− 17 days); $P < 0.001$.
- In-hospital mortality was higher in the standard group (29%) compared to the NPPV group (9%)

Criticisms and Limitations: The authors did not include an a priori power analysis with a stated benchmark for the expected rate of intubation in the study population. There was a very high rate of intubation (76%) in the standard therapy arm, raising questions about the management of patients in the control group.

Other Relevant Studies and Information:

- The investigators' conclusions are supported by other contemporaneous[2, 3] and subsequent randomized studies,[4, 5] as well as a meta-analysis of 14 randomized control trials.[6]
- NPPV has also been demonstrated to reduce the rate of intubation and improve mortality in patients with acute cardiogenic pulmonary edema.[7]

Summary and Implications: The trial by Brochard and colleagues[1] was the first large, multi-center, randomized controlled trial to demonstrate that the use of NPPV decreases the rate of endotracheal intubation, complications, length of hospital stay and in-hospital mortality among patients with acute

COPD exacerbations. Since the publication of this trial, the use of NPPV has been internationally adopted as the first-line intervention for respiratory failure due to acute COPD exacerbation and is now considered the standard of care.[8]

CLINICAL CASE: NONINVASIVE VENTILATION FOR ACUTE EXACERBATION OF COPD

Case History:

A 71-year-old man with hypertension and COPD on home nasal cannula oxygen at 2 L/min presents to the Emergency Department with acute dyspnea following several days of cough and increased sputum production. He denies fever, chest, or abdominal pain or any neurological symptoms. His respiratory rate is 33 breaths/min, heart rate 125 beats/min, blood pressure 170/93 mm Hg, and his oxygen saturation is 88% on nasal cannula oxygen at 4 L/min. He demonstrates increased work of breathing and has difficulty speaking in complete sentences. An arterial blood gas reveals a pH 7.20, $PaCO_2$ 90 mm Hg, PaO_2 60 mm Hg, and bicarbonate concentration 32 mmol/L.

How should this patient be treated?

Suggested Answer:

This patient has signs and symptoms of acute respiratory failure due to an acute COPD exacerbation. Unless the patient has a contraindication or cannot tolerate it, a trial of NPPV should be instituted immediately to improve respiratory symptoms and alveolar hypoventilation. During the trial of NPPV, further diagnostic studies can be completed, such as point-of-care ultrasound evaluation of his heart and lungs and chest radiography, while medical therapy is initiated with bronchodilators, corticosteroids, and antibiotics, if appropriate. Brochard and colleagues demonstrated that the use of NPPV in this setting reduces endotracheal intubation, complications of mechanical ventilation, hospital LOS, and mortality.[1]

References

1. Brochard L, Mancebo J, Wysocki M, et al. Noninvasive ventilation for acute exacerbations of chronic obstructive pulmonary disease. *New Engl J Med.* 1995; 333(13):817–822.

2. Bott J, Carroll MP, Conway JH, et al. Randomised controlled trial of nasal ventilation in acute ventilator failure due to chronic obstructive airways disease. *Lancet.* 1993; 341(8860):1555–1557.
3. Kramer N, Meyer TJ, Meharg J, Cece RD, Hill NS. Randomized, prospective trial of noninvasive positive pressure ventilation in acute respiratory failure. *Am J Respir Crit Care Med.* 1995;151(6):1799–1806.
4. Martin TJ, Hovis JD, Constantino JP, et al. A randomized, prospective evaluation of noninvasive ventilation for acute respiratory failure. *Am J Respir Crit Care Med.* 2000; 161:807–813.
5. Plant PK, Owen JL, Elliott MW. Early use of noninvasive ventilation for acute exacerbations of chronic obstructive pulmonary disease on general respiratory wards: a multicenter randomized controlled trial. *Lancet.* 2000; 355(9219):1931–1935.
6. Ram FS, Picot J, Lightowler J, Wedzicha JA. Noninvasive positive pressure ventilation for treatment of respiratory failure due to exacerbations of chronic obstructive pulmonary disease. *Cochrane Database Syst Rev.* 2004; (3): CD004104.
7. Masip J, Roque M, Sanchez B, Fernandez R, Subirana M, Exposito JA. Noninvasive ventilation in acute cardiogenic pulmonary edema: systematic review and meta-analysis. *JAMA.* 2005; 294:3124–3130.
8. Global Strategy for the Diagnosis, Management and Prevention of COPD. *Global Initiative for Chronic Obstructive Lung Disease (GOLD).* 2017. Available from: http://www.goldcopd.org/ Accessed 3/18/2017.

30

High-Frequency Oscillation in Early Acute Respiratory Distress Syndrome

SUSAN R. WILCOX AND HAITHAM S. AL ASHRY

"In adults with moderate to severe ARDS, the early application of HFOV targeting lung recruitment — as compared with a ventilation strategy that uses low tidal volume and high PEEP and that permits HFOV only in cases of refractory hypoxemia — does not reduce mortality and may be harmful.."

— FERGUSON ET AL, OSCILLATE Trial Investigators

Research Question: Does high-frequency oscillatory ventilation (HFOV) decrease mortality compared with conventional ventilation when applied early in patients with moderate to severe ARDS?[1]

Funding: The Canadian Institutes of Health Research, Randomized Controlled Trial (RCT) Program (Ottawa), and the King Abdullah International Medical Research Center (Riyadh, Saudi Arabia).

Year Study Began: 2007

Year Study Published: 2013

Study Location: 39 intensive care units in Canada, the United States, Saudi Arabia, Chile, and India

Who Was Studied: Patients with moderate to severe ARDS

Who Was Excluded: Patients with hypoxemia related to left atrial hypertension, pulmonary hemorrhage, neuromuscular disorders, severe chronic respiratory disease, preexisting conditions of expected 6-month mortality exceeding 50%, risk for intracranial hypertension, if the expected duration of mechanical ventilation was less than 48 hours, and those who were already receiving HFOV.

How Many Patients: The plan was to enroll 1200 patients, but the study was stopped after randomization of only 548 patients, based on an early signal of increased mortality in the HFOV group.

Study Overview: See Figure 30.1 for an overview of the study design.

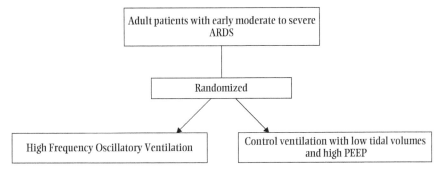

Figure 30.1 Summary of the study design.

Study Intervention: After enrollment, all patients received pressure ventilation to achieve a tidal volume of 6 mL per kilogram, and an FiO_2 of 0.60 with a PEEP level of 10 cm of water or higher if needed were provided for oxygenation. After 30 minutes, if the $PaO_2:FiO_2$ ratio was ≤ 200 the patients underwent randomization; otherwise the ventilator settings were maintained, and the patients were reassessed at least once daily for up to 72 hours.

For patients assigned to the HFOV group, a recruitment maneuver was first performed using a pressure of 40 cmH_2O for 40 seconds. HFOV was then initiated with a mean airway pressure (MAP) of 30 cmH_2O. The MAP and FiO_2 were increased per a predefined protocol[2] to target PaO_2 levels of 55 to 80 mm Hg. The highest possible frequency was used to minimize tidal volumes as long as pH was kept above 7.25. An inspiratory to expiratory ratio of 1:2 and pressure amplitude of 90 $cm\ H_2O$ were targeted. After 24 hours on the HFOV protocol, patients could be switched to the controlled ventilation protocol if they were able to be weaned to a MAP $\leq 24\ cmH_2O$ for 12 hours.

For patients assigned to the controlled ventilation group, a recruitment maneuver was performed (the same as that used for the HFOV group) and then a tidal volume of 6 mL/kg and a plateau pressure less than 35 cm H_2O were targeted. Initially a PEEP of 20 cmH_2O was used, then FiO_2 and PEEP were adjusted according to defined specified protocol. When patients were able to be weaned to FiO_2 of 0.4 and PEEP of 10 cm H_2O, there were no limits on tidal volumes or airway pressures.

Physicians were allowed to decrease the MAP or PEEP for patients in either group in the case of clinical or radiologic evidence of lung distension. For patients with persistent hypoxemia despite FiO_2 levels of 0.9, prone positioning or inhaled nitric oxide could be used. Alternative modes of ventilation including HFOV in the controlled ventilation group could be used in cases of refractory hypoxemia.

Follow-Up: Patients were followed until hospital discharge or death.

Endpoints: The primary outcome was the in hospital mortality. Secondary outcomes included: ICU mortality, 28-day mortality, and new barotrauma.

RESULTS

- More patients in the HFOV group received neuromuscular blockers than in the control group (83% vs. 68%, $P < 0.001$). In addition, more patients in the HFOV group received vasopressors (91% vs. 84%, $P = 0.01$) and received them for a longer period of time than in the control group (5 days vs. 3 days, $P = 0.01$).
- The doses of midazolam were higher in the HFOV group than the control group (199 mg per day vs. 141 mg per day, P value < 0.001). There was also a trend toward higher doses of opioids in the HFOV group.
- There was a trend toward increased barotrauma in the HFOV group compared with the control group (18% and 13%, $P = 0.13$).
- The use of renal replacement therapy, glucocorticoids, nitric oxide, prone positioning, and extra-corporeal support was similar in both arms (Table 30.1).

Table 30.1. SUMMARY OF THE STUDY KEY FINDINGS

Outcome	HFOV ($N = 275$)	Conventional ventilation ($N = 273$)	P value
In hospital mortality	129 (47%)	96 (35%)	0.005
ICU mortality	123 (45%)	84 (31%)	0.001
28 day mortality	111 (40%)	78 (29%)	0.004

Criticisms and Limitations:

- Early termination of the study may have resulted in overestimation of the harm in the HFOV arm. However, given the strong mortality signal, it is unlikely that HFOV could have exhibited survival benefit if the trial were completed.[3]
- The study used relatively high mean airway pressure; initial mean airway pressures were 30 cm H_2O and often increased up to 38 cm H_2O. These high intrathoracic pressures may have resulted in decreased preload and right ventricular dysfunction, and consequently hemodynamic compromise. Moreover, the high airway pressures used in the HFOV group may have led to increased barotrauma.[4] These differences may have masked any mortality benefit of HFOV.
- The study used central venous pressure greater than 12 cm H_2O as the cutoff point for adequate intravascular volume prior to initiating the study protocol. However, central venous pressure has been shown to be an imperfect surrogate for volume status and preload. Echocardiogram, pulse pressure variation, or other monitoring technologies should have been used for more accurate intravascular volume monitoring during HFOV.
- Systematic differences between the sedation strategies and frequency of neuromuscular blocking agents use in the two study groups may have confounded the study's findings.

Other Relevant Studies and Information:

- Prior studies comparing HFOV to conventional ventilation as an initial therapy for adult ARDS patients either used high tidal volumes in the conventional therapy arms or had small sample sizes.[5]
- The OSCAR multicenter trial randomized 795 patients who met established diagnostic criteria for ARDS and were expected to require ventilation for at least 2 days to either high frequency oscillatory ventilation (HFOV) or conventional ventilatory support. No statistically significant difference in 30-day mortality was observed between the patient cohorts. Furthermore, there was no significant difference between the groups for length of ICU and hospital stay, antibiotic use or vasopressors and inotropic support. Both OSCAR and OSCILLATE therefore contrast to previous meta-analysis suggesting benefit of HFOV in ARDS patients.[6]
- A recent metaanalysis of seven randomized controlled trials comparing HFOV with conventional lung-protective ventilation in acute respiratory distress syndrome found that the incidence of refractory hypoxemia

was significantly less with the use of HFOV. However HFOV was not associated with any in-hospital or 30-day mortality benefit.[7]

Summary and Implications: Early application of HFOV in moderate to severe ARDS patients does not result in survival benefit and may increase mortality.

CLINICAL CASE: EARLY APPLICATION OF HFOV IN MODERATE TO SEVERE ARDS PATIENTS

Case History:
A 55-year-old woman is admitted to the ICU with community acquired pneumonia. She is intubated due to significant respiratory distress hypoxemia. Chest x-ray shows bilateral air space opacities, and her PaO_2/FiO_2 is 120 on FiO_2 of 0.6. Based on the results of OSCILLATE study, what ventilation strategy should be used?

Suggested Answer:
OSCILLATE showed that HFOV may increase mortality when initiated early in moderate to severe ARDS patients. Therefore, a low tidal volume strategy using conventional ventilation should be used initially and the use of HFOV should be limited to salvage therapy.

References

1. Ferguson ND, Cook DJ, Guyatt GH, et al. High-frequency oscillation in early acute respiratory distress syndrome. *N Engl J Med.* 2013;368:795–805.
2. Fessler HE, Derdak S, Ferguson ND, et al. A protocol for high-frequency oscillatory ventilation in adults: results from a roundtable discussion. *Crit Care Med.* 2007;35:1649–1654.
3. Pocock SJ. When (not) to stop a clinical trial for benefit. *JAMA.* 2005; 294:2228–2230.
4. Guervilly C, Forel JM, Hraiech S, et al. Right ventricular function during high-frequency oscillatory ventilation in adults with acute respiratory distress syndrome. *Crit Care Med.* 2012;40:1539–1545.
5. Sud, S., Sud, M., Friedrich, J. O., et al. High frequency oscillation in patients with acute lung injury and acute respiratory distress syndrome (ARDS): systematic review and meta-analysis. *BMJ.* 2010;340:c2327.
6. Young D, Lamb SE, Shah S, et al; OSCAR Study Group. High-frequency oscillation for acute respiratory distress syndrome. *N Engl J Med.* 2013;368:806–813.
7. Maitra S, Bhattacharjee S, Khanna P, Baidya DK. High-frequency ventilation does not provide mortality benefit in comparison with conventional lung-protective ventilation in acute respiratory distress syndrome: a meta-analysis of the randomized controlled trials. *Anesthesiology.* 2015;122:841–851.

Gastrointestinal/Nutrition

31

Risk Factors for Gastrointestinal Bleeding in Critically Ill Patients

MIGUEL COBAS AND MELISSA GRILLO

"Our results support the use of prophylaxis in the subgroup of patients in the intensive care unit who have a coagulopathy or undergo mechanical ventilation for more than 48 hours."

—DJ COOK ET AL.

Research Question: Which critically ill patients are most likely to benefit from prophylaxis against stress ulcers to prevent GI bleeding?[1]

Funding: Ontario Ministry of Health

Year Study Began: 1990

Year Study Published: 1994

Study Location: Four university affiliated medical-surgical intensive care units in Ontario Canada

Who Was Studied: Consecutive patients more than 16 years of age who were hospitalized between June 1990 and July 1991.

Who Was Excluded: Patients with upper gastrointestinal bleeding within 48 hours before or 24 hours after admission, previous total gastrectomy, facial trauma or epistaxis, brain death, a hopeless prognosis or either death or discharge within 24 hours after admission.

How Many Patients: 2252

Study Overview: A prospective multicenter cohort study was conducted evaluating potential risk factors for stress ulcers in ICU patients. The 12 potential risk factors evaluated daily were sepsis, hypotension, renal failure, coagulopathy, hepatic failure, Glasgow coma score less than 5, anticoagulant therapy, glucocorticoid administration, nonsteroidal anti-inflammatory drug administration, respiratory failure, the use of active enteral feeding, and the use of two or more doses of stress ulcer prophylaxis. The occurrence of clinically important gastrointestinal bleeding was documented. Attending physicians were encouraged to withhold prophylaxis against stress ulcers in all patients except those with head injury, burns over more than 30% of BSA, organ transplants, and diagnosis of peptic ulcer disease or gastritis in the preceding six weeks or upper GI bleeding three days to six weeks before admission. Prophylaxis was defined as the administration of two or more doses of histamine H2 receptor antagonists, antacid, sucralfate, prostaglandin analogs, or omeprazole (Figure 31.1).

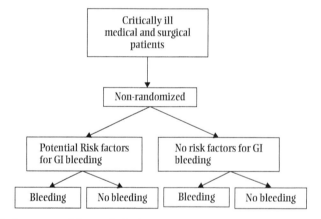

Figure 31.1 Summary of the study design.

Endpoints: Overt bleeding and clinically important gastrointestinal bleeding. Overt bleeding was defined as hematemesis, gross blood or "coffee grounds" material in nasogastric aspirate, hematochezia, or melena. Clinically important bleeding was defined as overt bleeding complicated by one of the following within twenty four hours after onset of bleeding: a spontaneous decrease of more than twenty mm Hg in the systolic blood pressure, an increase of more than 20 beats per minute in the heart rate, a decrease of more than 10 mm Hg in the systolic blood pressure measured on sitting up, or a decrease in the hemoglobin level of more than 2 grams per deciliter and subsequent transfusion.

RESULTS

- Of 2252 patients, 674 received prophylaxis against stress ulcers. One hundred patients had overt bleeding (4.4%), 87 of which were receiving prophylaxis. Thirty-three patients (1.5%) had clinically important bleeding and of these 23 were receiving prophylaxis.
- The source of bleeding was identified in 22 of the 33 patients who had important bleeding, being the most common gastric and duodenal ulcers (11) and gastric erosions (8).
- Independent risk factors for clinically important bleeding identified in the multiple regression analysis were respiratory failure requiring mechanical ventilation for more than 48 hours (odds ratio 15.6) and coagulopathy (odds ratio 4.3). These two factors were predictive regardless of whether the patient was receiving prophylaxis or not.
- Of 847 patients at high risk (those with respiratory failure or coagulopathy), thirty-one had clinically important bleeding (3.7%).
- Of the 1405 patients at low risk, only two had clinically important bleeding (0.1%) (Table 31.1).

Table 31.1. CLINICALLY IMPORTANT GASTROINTESTINAL BLEEDING AMONG 2252 PATIENTS ADMITTED TO AN INTENSIVE CARE UNIT, ACCORDING TO THE PRESENCE OR ABSENCE OF RESPIRATORY FAILURE AND COAGULOPATHY

Patient Group and Risk Factor	Percentage with Bleeding
All Patients	
Neither	0.1
Respiratory failure	2.0
Coagulopathy	0.5
Both	8.4
Total	1.5
Patients who received prophylaxis	
Neither	0.4
Respiratory failure	3.7
Coagulopathy	0.0
Both	9.8
Total	3.43
Patients who did not receive prophylaxis	
Neither	0.1
Respiratory failure	0.9
Coagulopathy	0.8
Both	6.1
Total	0.6

Adapted from Cook DJ, Fuller HD, Guyatt GH, et al.; Canadian Critical Care Trials Group. Risk factors for gastrointestinal bleeding in critically ill patients. *N Engl J Med* 1994; 330:377–381.

Criticisms and Limitations:

- The study did not clearly indicate how critically ill patients should be identified and almost half were cardiovascular surgical patients—a group at low risk for stress ulcer complications.
- There were low rates of sepsis (1.6%), cardiovascular (6.3%), or respiratory disease (12.1%) as indication for ICU admission in the study population which might impact the generalizability.
- Coagulopathy might better be defined by an elevation in fibrin-split products or thromboelastogram abnormalities rather than alterations in PT/aPTT as therapeutic anticoagulation (e.g., warfarin and heparin) do not increase risk for GI bleeding.

Other Relevant Studies and Information:

- The incidence of clinically significant GI bleeding has steadily decreased over the last few decades. The reason for this decrease is likely a combination of overall improved care in the ICU, aggressive treatment of hypotension, and the earlier initiation of enteral feedings.[2]
- Several meta-analyses and cost-effectiveness studies suggest proton pump inhibitors (PPIs) to be more clinically effective for stress ulceration prophylaxis in critically ill patients histamine-2 receptor antagonists.[3]
- Although the vast majority of patients in ICUs receive stress-ulcer prophylaxis, largely with PPIs, some controversy surrounds their efficacy and safety. Some reports suggest that the use of PPIs increases the risk of nosocomial infections, orthopedic fractures, medication interactions, and malabsorption syndromes.[4]
- A 2010 meta-analysis demonstrated no benefit from stress ulcer prophylaxis when added to enteric feedings.[5] A recent randomized controlled trial found we found no evidence that the prophylactic administration of pantoprazole is of benefit for or is harmful to mechanically ventilated critically ill patients who were expected to receive enteral nutrition.[4]

Summary and Implications: The study's most important finding is that simple clinical criteria (i.e., respiratory failure requiring mechanical ventilation for more than 48 hours and coagulopathy) can be used to predict which ICU patients have the highest risk of bleeding from stress ulceration. This finding allows more selective use of stress ulcer prophylaxis thereby avoiding unnecessary exposure of patients to the potential side effects of prophylaxis and reducing cost. Based on the study findings, the number of patients needed to treat to prevent a single episode of bleeding is very high (900 patients), making the case that in low risk patients, prophylaxis can be safely withheld.

CLINICAL CASE: STRESS ULCER PROPHYLAXIS IN THE CRITICALLY ILL

Case History:

A 27-year-old male, who sustained an isolated splenic laceration in a motor vehicle accident, is admitted to the ICU after undergoing an exploratory laparotomy and splenectomy. He has no clinical evidence of coagulopathy, his platelet count is 150,000, and his PT and PTT are within normal limits. Should stress ulcer prophylaxis be initiated?

Suggested Answer:

Few critically ill patients experience clinically significant gastrointestinal bleeding from stress ulceration. The study by Cook et al. identified two independent risk factors for gastrointestinal bleeding in the critically ill: mechanical ventilation greater than 48 hours and coagulopathy.[1] This patient had an isolated splenic injury and is likely to be extubation within 48 hours and has no evidence of coagulopathy. Thus, prophylaxis can safely be withheld.

References

1. Cook DJ, Fuller HD, Guyatt GH, et al.; Canadian Critical Care Trials Group. Risk factors for gastrointestinal bleeding in critically ill patients. *N Engl J Med* 1994; 330:377–381.
2. Marik PE, Vasu T, Hirani A, Pachinburavan M. Stress ulcer prophylaxis in the new millennium: a systematic review and meta-analysis. *Crit Care Med.* 2010;38(11):2222–2228.
3. Alhazzani W, Alenezi F, Jaeschke RZ, et al. Proton pump inhibitors versus histamine 2 receptor antagonists for stress ulcer prophylaxis in critically ill patients: a systematic review and meta-analysis. *Crit Care Med.* 2013;41(3):693–705.
4. MacLaren R, Reynolds PM, Allen RR. Histamine-2 receptor antagonists vs. proton pump inhibitors on gastrointestinal tract hemorrhage and infectious complications in the intensive care unit. *JAMA Intern Med.* 2014;174(4):564–574.
5. Selvanderan SP, Summers MJ, Finnis ME, et al. Pantoprazole or placebo for stress ulcer prophylaxis (POP-UP): randomized double-blind exploratory study. *Crit Care Med.* 2016;44(10):1842–1850.

32

Early versus Late Parenteral Nutrition in the ICU

The EPaNIC (Early Parenteral Nutrition Completing Enteral Nutrition in Adult Critically Ill Patients) Trial

D. DANTE YEH

"Late initiation of parenteral nutrition was associated with faster recovery and fewer complications, as compared with early initiation."
—THE EPaNIC INVESTIGATOR

Research Question: At what time point should ICU patients unable to achieve sufficient nutrition via enteral nutrition (EN) be started on supplemental parenteral nutrition (SPN)?[1]

Funding: Methusalem program of the Flemish government, the Research Fund of the Catholic University of Leuven, the Research Foundation Flanders, Clinical Research Fund of the University Hospitals Leuven, and Baxter Healthcare.

Year Began: 2007

Year Study Published: 2011

Study Location: 7 ICUs in Belgium

Who Was Studied: Adults admitted to an ICU who were nutritionally at risk (nutritional risk screening [NRS] score ≥ 3)

Who Was Excluded: Patients under age 18, those who were moribund or coded DNR, those enrolled in another trial, those with short-bowel syndrome, those on home ventilation, those in a diabetic coma, those already on a nutritional regimen when referred, those who were pregnant or lactating, those without a central catheter, those already taking oral nutrition, those who had been readmitted to ICU, those with a body mass index (BMI) ≤ 17, and those with a Nutrition Risk Screening 2002 (NRS 2002) score < 3.

How Many Patients: 4640

Study Overview: Using a randomized design, this study compared the effect of late initiation of parenteral nutrition (American and Canadian guidelines) with early initiation (ESPEN guidelines) on complication rates and mortality in adult ICU patients who were nutritionally at risk but who were not chronically malnourished (body mass index ≥17). Since all the participating ICUs followed the guidelines for early initiation of parenteral nutrition, the active intervention was late initiation (Figure 32.1).

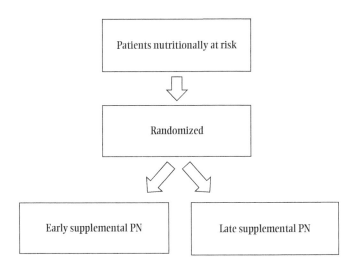

Figure 32.1 Summary of the study design.

Study Intervention: Patients in the early-initiation group received intravenous (IV) glucose (20%) starting immediately and targeting 400 kcal on ICU day 1 and 800 kcal on ICU day 2. On the third ICU day, SPN was started with the goal to deliver 100% of caloric goal using combined enteral and parenteral nutrition.

Patients in the late-initiation group received IV 5% dextrose in a volume equal to the early-initiation group (to provide adequate hydration) for the first week of ICU stay. If enteral nutrition was insufficient (<80% of calculated caloric goal), SPN was started on day 8.

In both groups, SPN was reduced and eventually stopped when EN provided ≥80% of caloric target or when the patient was able to begin oral intake. SPN was resumed when enteral or oral intake was <50% of caloric target. All patients were maintained semi-recumbent, maintained tight glycemic control (target blood glucose level 80 to 100mg/dL), and had protocolized use of prokinetic agents and duodenal feeding tubes.

Follow-Up: 90 days after enrollment

Endpoints: Primary safety endpoints: rates of survival (proportion of patients alive at discharge from the ICU in ≤ 8 days, rates of ICU and hospital death, rates of survival up to 90 days) and rates of complications and hypoglycemia. Primary efficacy endpoint: duration of dependency on intensive care (defined as number of ICU days and time to readiness for discharge from the ICU). Secondary efficacy endpoints: new infections, duration of mechanical ventilation, tracheostomy, acute kidney injury, liver dysfunction, duration of hospital stay, functional status, and health care costs.

RESULTS

- There were similar rates of death in the ICU, hospital, and at 90 days. Although there were higher rates of hypoglycemia in the late-initiation group (3.5% vs. 1.9%, $p = 0.001$), the proportion of patients discharged alive from the ICU within 8 days was higher in the late vs. early initiation group (75.2% vs. 71.7%, $p = 0.007$). All other complications were similar between the groups.
- The late-initiation group had a median stay in the ICU that was 1 day shorter than in the early-initiation group
- The late-initiation group had lower rate of new infections, shorter duration of mechanical ventilation, and shorter duration of renal-replacement therapy
- The late-initiation group had shorter duration of hospitalization by 2 days. Functional status at hospital discharge (6-minute walk distance and activities of daily living) was similar between groups. The late-initiation group had lower mean total health care costs.
- Predefined subgroups (BMI <25 or ≥ 40 or NRS ≥ 5; cardiac surgery; sepsis) analyses showed no heterogeneity and confirmed the overall trends.

Criticisms and Limitations: First, the parenteral nutrition solution did not contain glutamine nor other immune-modulating agents (such as fish oils). However, these pharmaconutrients are not in routine use in most ICUs and furthermore, their use is controversial. Second, because the PN was premixed and standardized, they had a relatively low protein-to-calorie ratio. The vast majority received less than 1g/kg/day of protein for the entire duration of the study, which is far less than the 1.5–2.0 g/kg/day currently recommended for critically ill adults. There is accumulating evidence that sufficient protein intake may be more important than sufficient calorie intake for clinically important outcomes.[2] Third, the caloric target was calculated using standard equations based on corrected body weight. Routine indirect calorimetry (IC), currently considered the gold standard, was not used. However, because IC is not routinely used in the majority of ICUs worldwide, this "limitation" increases the generalizability of the results. Finally, while the group assignments were unblinded, the endpoints were objective, limiting the potential for bias.

Additional Limitations:

- The majority (~75%) of the patients had a BMI 20–30, and their conclusions may not be valid in obese patients
- Less than half of the enrolled patients were classified as "Emergency admission" and over 60% were post-cardiac surgery. This patient mix limits the generalizability of the study.
- The overall median ICU duration was only 3 days. Although they had moderate APACHE II scores (23), it is unclear how truly "sick" they were if they needed only a short ICU stay. The low acuity is reflected by the fact that the overall mortality was only about 6%. Additionally, nutritional management *after* ICU discharge was at the discretion of the attending physician.

Other Relevant Studies and Information: In a follow-up study, the authors reported on a subgroup of EPaNIC patients undergoing serial CT scans. This analysis demonstrated that early-initiation of PN resulted in *reduced quality of muscle tissue* (as evidenced by increased lipid conversion).[3] This was corroborated clinically in another follow-up study reporting that more patients in the early-initiation PN group developed ICU-acquired weakness.[4]

Based on this and other studies, guidelines from the Society of Critical Care Medicine and the American Society of Parenteral and Enteral Nutrition recommend that "in the patient at low nutrition risk (e.g., NRS 2002 ≤ 3), exclusive PN be withheld over the first 7 days following ICU admission if the patient cannot maintain volitional intake and if early EN is not feasible."[5]

Summary and Implications: In this study involving relatively thin patients with short ICU stays who were receiving tight glycemic control, early parenteral nutrition (3 days) did not result in lower rates of mortality vs. late parenteral nutrition (8 days), despite delivering significantly more calories in the first ICU week. In fact, late initiation of parenteral nutrition was associated with a shorter duration of mechanical ventilation, a lower incidence of renal replacement therapy, a lower incidence of infections, and a shorter ICU and hospital length of stay. Despite its criticisms, the EPaNIC study provides strong evidence favoring late PN in this patient population.

CLINICAL CASE: EARLY VERSUS LATE PARENTERAL NUTRITION

Case History:

A 76-year-old woman on warfarin for atrial fibrillation tripped and fell down a flight of stairs, resulting in a moderate traumatic brain injury requiring intubation for airway protection. Additional injuries include multiple rib fractures, Grade 1 splenic laceration, multiple lumbar transverse process fractures, a type 1 odontoid fracture, and a non-displaced tibia/fibula fracture. Her BMI is 19 (wt = 50 kg) and her daughter reports that in the past month she has not been eating well and she has lost about 7 pounds.

Upon arrival in the ICU, an orogastric tube is placed and enteral nutrition is started. However, she has frequent interruptions for CT scans and high gastric residual volumes > 500 mL. A central line was placed for infusion of hyperosmolar therapy and vasopressor support to maximize cerebral perfusion pressure. On ICU day 3, she vomits while on "trophic" tube feeds. Based on the results of EPaNIC, how should this patient be treated?

Suggested Answer:

EPaNIC showed that late-initiation of supplemental PN resulted in faster recovery and fewer complications when compared to early-initiation. The patient in the vignette is at high nutritional risk for multiple reasons (age, severity of disease, impaired baseline nutritional status), and it is tempting to attempt to provide aggressive nutritional therapy using a mixed (EN + PN) approach. However, infusing calories intravenously may harm this patient and prolong her mechanical ventilation, ICU, and hospital stay. This patient should remain semi-recumbent and prokinetic therapy should be initiated to facilitate gastric emptying. For the first week of ICU stay, efforts should be maximized to deliver enteral nutrition to reach her caloric target. If these efforts remain unsuccessful at ICU day 8, then supplemental PN would be an appropriate next step.

References

1. Casaer et al. Early versus late parenteral nutrition in critically ill adults. *N Engl J Med.* 2011;365:506–517.
2. Nicolo M, Heyland DK, Chittams J, et al. Clinical outcomes related to protein delivery in a critically ill population: a multicenter, multinational observation study. *JPEN.* 2016;40(1):45–51.
3. Casaer MP et al. Impact of early parenteral nutrition on muscle and adipose tissue compartments during critical illness. *Crit Care Med.* 2013;41(10):2298–2309.
4. Hermans et al. Effect of tolerating macronutrient deficit on the development of intensive-care unit acquired weakness: a subanalysis of the EPaNIC trial. *Lancet Respir Med.* 2013;1(8):621–629.
5. McClave et al. Guidelines for the provision and assessment of nutrition support therapy in the adult critically ill patient: Society of Critical Care Medicine (SCCM) and American Society for Parenteral and Enteral Nutrition (A.S.P.E.N.). *JPEN.* 2016; 40(2):159–211.

33

Initial Trophic versus Full Enteral Feeding in Patients with Acute Lung Injury

The EDEN Randomized Trial

MILAD SHARIFPOUR AND PEDRO MENDEZ-TELLEZ

"In patients with acute lung injury, compared with full enteral feeding, a strategy of initial trophic enteral feeding for up to 6 days did not improve ventilator free days, 60-day mortality, or infectious complications but was associated with less gastrointestinal intolerance."

—RICE ET AL.

Research Question: In patients with acute lung injury (ALI) and without malnutrition does trophic enteral feeding during the first 6 days of critical illness increase ventilator-free days (VFDs) and decrease gastrointestinal intolerance compared with full enteral feeding?[1]

Sponsor: National Heart, Lung, and Blood Institute Acute Respiratory Distress Syndrome (ARDS) Clinical Trials Network (ARDSNet).

Year Study Began: 2008

Year Study Published: 2012

Study Location: 44 hospitals in the National Heart, Lung, and Blood Institute ARDS Clinical Trials Network.

Who Was Studied: Adult patients with no obvious malnutrition, within 48 hours of ALI onset, who receiving mechanical ventilation for less than 72 hours. ALI was defined by the ratio of the partial pressure of arterial oxygen (PaO_2) to the fraction of inspired oxygen (FiO_2) of less than 300, with evidence of bilateral pulmonary infiltrates on chest x-ray, consistent with pulmonary edema, without clinical evidence of elevated left atrial pressure.

Who Was Excluded: Patients with chronic lung diseases, those outside of the ALI time window, those who had received mechanical ventilation for > 72 hours at the time of randomization, patients with severe liver disease or fatal underlying diseases, patients with refractory shock, intracranial hemorrhage, severe neuro-muscular diseases, or severe malnutrition, or moribund patients.

How Many Patients: 1,000 patients were randomized.

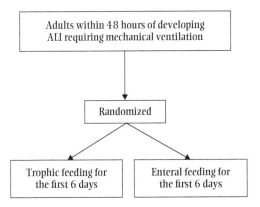

Figure 33.1 Summary of the study design.

Study Overview: See Figure 33.1 for an overview of the study design.

Study Interventions: Participants were randomized to receive either trophic (~25% of target caloric requirements) or full enteral feeding within 6 hours of randomization, for the first 6 days of the study. In patients randomized to initial low volume enteral feeding tube feeds were started at 10 mL/h (10 20 kcal/h). This trial was part of a 2 x 2 factorial trial design, where patients were also randomized to Omega-3 fatty acids (OMEGA study) or a control solution. The first 272 patients received omega-3 or control supplement (total of 240 mL/day). Once administration of omega-3 supplements was stopped, feeding rates were increased to 20 kcal/h to approximate the calories provided by omega-3 supplements. Gastric residual volumes (GRVs) were checked every 12 hours.

In patients randomized to full feeding group, enteral feeds were started at 25 mL/h and advanced to goal rates (of ~80 kcal/h) as quickly as possible. GRVs were checked every 6 hours while increasing feeding rates. Full feeding rates were calculated with the goal of providing 25–30 kcal/kg/day of non-protein calories and 1.2–1.6 g/kg/day of protein.

Both the trophic and full feeding strategies specified when and for how long to hold enteral nutrition for elevated GRVs (greater than 400 mL), and for other gastrointestinal intolerances. After 6 days, the patients randomized to initial trophic feeding were advanced to full enteral feeding if they were still receiving mechanical ventilation.

Follow-Up: 90 days.

Endpoints: The two primary endpoints were the number of VFDs and mortality before hospital discharge. Secondary endpoints included the incidence of ventilator-associated pneumonia, percentage of goal enteral feeding, frequency of gastrointestinal intolerances, 60-day mortality before hospital discharge with unassisted breathing, ICU-free and organ failure– free days, and new infections.

RESULTS

Despite the full enteral feeding group receiving significantly more calories (1300 vs. 400 kcals/d), there were no differences in important clinical outcomes:

- VFDs to day 28 were not different between the trophic and full feeding groups 4.9 vs. 15.0, $p = 0.89$.
- There was no difference between the two groups in 60-day mortality 23.2% vs. 22.2, $p = 0.77$.
- There were no differences between the two groups in organ failure-free days, ICU-free days, or the incidence of new infections.
- Participants receiving full enteric feedings had a higher incidence of gastrointestinal intolerance (regurgitation, vomiting, high gastric

residual volumes, and constipation) and higher need for antidiarrheal, or prokinetic agents Table 33.1).

Table 33.1. SUMMARY OF THE STUDY'S KEY FINDINGS

Outcome	Trophic feeding (n=508)	Full Feeding (n=492)	P Value
Ventilator-free days, No. (95% CI)	14.9 (13.9 – 15.6)	15.0 (14.1 – 15.9)	0.89
Failure-free days, No. (95% CI)			
Cardiovascular	19.1 (18.2 – 20.0)	18.9 (18.1 – 19.8)	0.75
Renal	20.0 (19.0 – 20.9)	19.4 (18.4 – 20.5)	0.43
Hepatic	22.0 (21.2 – 22.9)	22.6 (21.8 – 23.5)	0.37
Coagulation	22.3 (21.4 – 23.1)	23.1 (22.3 – 23.9)	0.16
ICU-free days, No. (95% CI)	14.3 (13.5 – 15.3)	14.7 (13.8 – 15.6)	0.67
60-d mortality, No. (%) [95% CI]	118 (23.2) [19.6–26.9]	109 (22.2) [18.5–25.8]	0.77
Development of infections, No. (%)[95%]			
VAP	37 (7.3) [5.0–9.5]	33 (6.7) [4.5–8.9]	0.72
Clostridium difficile colitis	15 (3.0) [1.5–4.4]	13 (2.6) [1.2–4.1]	0.77
Bacteremia, No. (%)	59 (11.6) [8.8–14.4]	46 (9.3) [6.8–11.9]	0.24

Criticisms and Limitations:

- The open label study design introduces potential bias in the reporting of gastrointestinal intolerance. GRVs were checked twice as frequently in the full feeding group.
- Almost 90% of the screened patients were excluded, which may limit the generalizability of the results.
- The majority of the patients in the study came from adult medical ICUs therefore it is unclear whether the study results are generalizable to surgical patients.
- Malnourished and underweight patients were excluded. This study provides no information regarding the risks (e.g. refeeding

syndrome) or benefits of early nutrition in patients with malnutrition.

- Patients did not receive concomitant parenteral nutrition therefore this study does not provide any information regarding the role of parenteral nutrition in patients with ALI.
- 60-day mortality might have been underestimated as it was assumed that patients discharged home without breathing assistance prior to day 60 were still alive at day 60.

Other Relevant Studies and Information: Two follow-up studies to the EDEN trial evaluated the effects of initial trophic feeding versus full energy enteral feeding on long-term physical and cognitive outcomes in patients with ALI. These studies found that as a group the patients with ALI had substantial physical, psychological, and cognitive impairments, reduced quality of life, and impaired return to work, at 6 and 12 months, with no difference between the two groups based on feeding strategy.[2, 3]

Summary and Implications: In a highly selected group of ALI patients, early trophic (hypocaloric) enteral feeding for up to 6 days was not associated with worse clinical outcomes compared to full enteral feeding. Additionally, this study suggested that many patients, including those in shock (40% of the patients), can be safely fed via a nasogastric tube (post pyloric feeding was used in less than 20% of patients), and that tolerating gastric residual volumes of up to 400 mL did not increase the rate of aspiration or ventilator induced pneumonia. It was also shown that protocolized feeding allows for delivering a higher percentage of the target caloric requirement.

CLINICAL CASE: INITIATING ENTERAL TUBE FEEDING IN PATIENTS WITH ACUTE RESPIRATORY DISTRESS SYNDROME

Case History:
You are the attending intensivist in the medical ICU. During morning rounds your intern suggests initiating enteral feeds for a 45-year-old previously well-nourished patient who was intubated 24 hours ago for ARDS secondary to community acquired pneumonia. Based on the results of this study, do you recommend initiating trophic feeds or full enteral feeds? Is it necessary to obtain postpyloric enteral access? Should you routinely monitor gastric residual volumes?

Suggested Answer:

This study suggests that initiation of early trophic (hypocaloric) enteral nutrition for up to 6 days is safe and is not associated with increased 60-day mortality, infectious complications, or length of stay or VFDs as compared to full enteral nutrition. Furthermore, this study showed that a majority of patients can be safely fed via a nasogastric tube, without requiring a postpyloric feeding tube.

Based on the results of the EDEN trial, trophic feeds via nasogastric tube can be safely initiated and continued for up to 6 days without increasing the risk of adverse outcomes. While the study does not directly address the question regarding routine GRV monitoring, it suggests that tolerating GRVs up to 400 mL may not increase the risk of aspiration or ventilator associated pneumonia.

References

1. Rice TW, Wheeler AP, Thompson BT, et al. Initial trophic vs full enteral feeding in patients with acute lung injury: the EDEN randomized trial. *JAMA*. 2012; 307(8):795–803.
2. Needham DM, Dinglas VD, Bienvenu OJ, et al. One-year outcomes in patients with acute lung injury randomized to initial trophic or full enteral feeding; prospective follow-up of EDEN randomized trial. *BMJ*. 2013; 346:f1532.
3. Needham, DM, Dinglas VD, Morris PE, et al. Physical and cognitive performance of patients with acute lung injury 1 year after initial trophic versus full enteral feeding. EDEN trial follow-up. *Am J Respir Crit Care Med*. 2013; 188(5):567–576.

Early versus On-Demand Nasoenteric Tube Feeding in Acute Pancreatitis

PETER J. FAGENHOLZ

"This trial did not show the superiority of early nasoenteric tube feeding as compared with an oral diet after 72 hours, in reducing the rate of infection or death in patients with acute pancreatitis at high risk for complications."

—BAKKER ET AL.

Research Question: Can rates of major infection and death in patients with severe acute pancreatitis be reduced by starting nasojejunal tube feeding within 24 hours?[1]

Sponsor: The Netherlands Organization for Health Research and Development

Year Study Began: 2008

Year Study Published: 2014

Study Location: 6 university medical centers and 13 large teaching hospitals in the Netherlands

Who Was Studied: Patients with a first episode of acute pancreatitis at any of the 19 teaching hospitals affiliated with the Dutch Pancreatitis Study Group. Patients were required to be at high risk of complications based on meeting any of the following criteria: (1) an Acute Physiology and Chronic Health Evaluation (APACHE) II score of 8 or higher, (2) an Imrie or modified Glasgow score of 3 or higher, or (3) a C-reactive protein level over 150 mg/L.

Who Was Excluded: Patients with post ERCP pancreatitis, malignancy-induced pancreatitis, patients with enteral or parenteral nutrition at home, pregnant patients, patients evaluated more than 24 hours after presentation to the emergency department, and patients presenting to the emergency department more than 96 hours after symptom onset were excluded.

How Many Patients: 208 patients were enrolled.

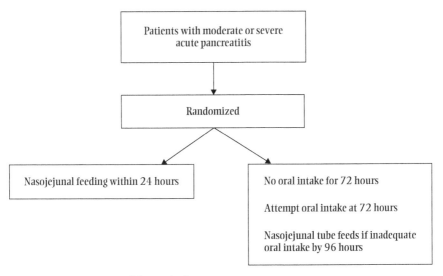

Figure 34.1 Summary of the study design.

Study Overview: See Figure 34.1 for an overview of the study design.

Study Intervention: Once patients were found to be eligible and consented, they were randomized to either the "early tube feeding" group, or the "on-demand tube feeding" group. The early tube feeding group underwent nasojejunal tube placement followed by initiation of nasojejunal tube feeding within 24 hours of randomization. The on-demand tube feeding group was started on an oral diet after 72 hours. If an oral diet was not tolerated by 96 hours, then a nasojejunal tube was placed and tube feeding was initiated.

Follow-Up: 6 months

Endpoints: The primary endpoint was a composite endpoint of major infection (infected pancreatic necrosis, bacteremia, or pneumonia) or death. Secondary endpoints included the development of necrotizing pancreatitis and the development of organ failure after randomization.

RESULTS

There was no difference between the groups with regard to the primary or secondary outcomes (Table 34.1).

Table 34.1. SUMMARY OF THE STUDY'S KEY FINDINGS

Outcome	Early Tube Feeding	On-Demand Tube Feeding	P Value
Major infection	25%	26%	0.87
Death	11%	7%	0.33
Multiple organ failure	10%	8%	0.77

Criticisms and Limitations:

- The study may have been underpowered to demonstrate significant differences based on nutritional strategy. Although the investigators tried to select patients at risk for significant complications of acute pancreatitis, only about 1/3 developed organ failure and an even lower percentage developed necrosis. Since the benefits of early feeding for reducing the risk of death or infectious complications in pancreatitis would be expected to be most pronounced in the sickest patients, dilution of the study population with patients having lower severity of illness might mask the benefit.
- Existing guidelines recommended using nasogastric tube feeding for patients with acute pancreatitis receiving enteral nutritional supplementation, reserving nasojejunal feeding for patients who do not tolerate nasogastric feeding. This guideline was not followed in this study[2]
- The timing of enteral nutrition initiation differed only modestly between the groups, with initiation occurring within 24 hours for the "early tube feeding" group versus 72 hours for an oral diet or 96 hours for tube feeding in the "on-demand tube feeding" group. This difference may have been too small to impact outcomes.

Other Relevant Studies and Information: The most recent guidelines from the American Pancreatic Association and International Association of Pancreatology, published after this trial, recommend feeding with either nasogastric or nasojejunal tube feeding.[3] The guidelines do not recommend a hard time or exact criteria for initiating enteral tube feeding, but cite a randomized controlled trial showing improved outcomes when enteral nutrition was begun within 48 hours of presentation compared to after 7 days of fasting.[4] It is already known that "on demand" feeding even with a regular diet initiated as soon as pain and inflammatory markers are improving is safe and can reduce length of stay in mild pancreatitis.[5]

Summary and Implications: There appears to be no benefit to routine early initiation of nasojejunal tube feeding compared to a strategy of waiting 72 hours and attempting oral intake. This may be particularly true in less severe acute pancreatitis when there is some expense and discomfort to tube feeding and there may be no benefit. Overall this study and the preponderance of data from other studies support an "on-demand" feeding strategy rather than early tube feeding, and to initiate this "on demand" oral feeding regimen somewhere within the 24–72-hour window. Initiating tube feeding by 96 hours in patients with inadequate oral intake is reasonable.

Early feeding and any resulting improvement in gut mucosal integrity may not be as important as previously thought for reducing infection and death in acute pancreatitis.

CLINICAL CASE: NUTRITION IN ACUTE PANCREATITIS

Case History:
A 55-year-old woman presents to the emergency department with epigastric pain, nausea, and vomiting. Serum amylase and lipase are elevated to greater than 10 times normal and C-reactive protein is 200 mg/L. She is hemodynamically stable and is admitted to the hospital ward for pain control, fluid resuscitation, and clinical observation. What is the best nutritional strategy for this patient?

Suggested Answer:
Based on this trial we should not place a nasojejunal tube and begin administering tube feeding within 24 hours. As a negative trial, it does not explicitly support the alternative study strategy either—denying oral or enteral nutrition for 72 hours before allowing on-demand feeding. Based on this study and the other available data discussed previously, the currently recommended nutritional strategy would be to wait until pain and markers of inflammation have begun to improve, and initiate an on-demand oral feeding regimen at that point. In patients not meeting nutritional goals by 96 hours after presentation, nasoenteric feeding should be begun. Parenteral nutrition should be reserved for patients not meeting nutritional goals by an enteral route 7 days after presentation.

References

1. Bakker OJ, van Brunschot S, van Santvoort HC, et. al. Early versus on-demand naso-enteric tube feeding in acute pancreatitis. *N Engl J Med.* 2014;371(21):1983–1993.
2. Meier R, Ockenga J, Pertkiewicz M, Pap A, Milinic N, Macfie J; DGEM (German Society for Nutritional Medicine), Löser C, Keim V; ESPEN (European Society for Parenteral and Enteral Nutrition). ESPEN guidelines on enteral nutrition: pancreas. *Clin Nutr.* 2006;25(2):275–284.
3. Working Group IAP/APA Acute Pancreatitis Guidelines. IAP/APA evidence-based guidelines for the management of acute pancreatitis. *Pancreatology.* 2013;13(4 Suppl 2): e1–15.
4. Moraes JM, Felga GE, Chebli LA, et al. A full solid diet as the initial meal in mild acute pancreatitis is safe and result in a shorter length of hospitalization: results from a prospective, randomized, controlled, double-blind clinical trial. *J Clin Gastroenterol.* 2010;44:517e22.
5. Sun JK, Mu XW, Li WQ, Tong ZH, Li J, Zheng SY. Effects of early enteral nutrition on immune function of severe acute pancreatitis patients. *World J Gastroenterol.* 2013;19(6):917–22.

35

Glutamine and Antioxidants in Critically Ill Patients

The REDOXS Trial

YUK MING LIU AND JARONE LEE

"Early provision of glutamine or antioxidants did not improve clinical outcomes, and glutamine was associated with an increase in mortality among critically ill patients with multiorgan failure."
—THE REDOXS INVESTIGATORS

Research Question: Does supplementation with glutamine and/or antioxidants improve 28-day mortality for critically ill patients?[1]

Funding: Canadian Institutes of Health Research and Fresenius Kabi

Year Study Began: 2005

Year Study Published: 2013

Study Location: 40 intensive care units in Canada, United States and Europe

Who Was Studied: Mechanically ventilated adult patients who were critically ill with multisystem organ failure. Two or more of the following organ failures related to the acute illness were included: acute lung injury, vasopressor agent requirement, renal dysfunction or thrombocytopenia.

Who Was Excluded: Patients who were >24 hours from admission to ICU, not expected to survive greater than 48 hours, anticipated withdrawal of care, absolute contraindications to enteral nutrition, severe traumatic brain injury, seizure disorder requiring anticonvulsant, Class C cirrhosis, metastatic cancer or Stage 4 lymphoma with < 6 month life expectancy, routine elective cardiac cases, burn patients > 30% body surface area, pregnant or lactating patients

How Many Patients: 1218

Study Overview: See Figure 35.1 for an overview of the study design.

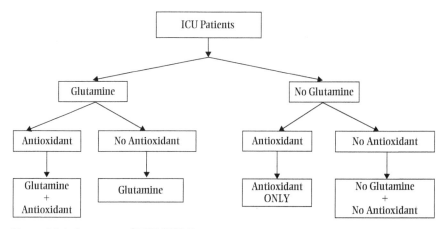

Figure 35.1 Summary of REDOXS Design.

Study Intervention: Using a 2 x 2 factorial design, patients were randomly assigned to receive glutamine supplementation or matching placebo solutions. In addition, patients were randomly assigned to receive selenium intravenously plus the following vitamins and minerals enterally: selenium, zinc, beta carotene, vitamin E and vitamin C.

Follow-up: Patients were followed for 6 months to determine survival rates.

Endpoints: Primary outcome was 28-day mortality. Secondary outcomes included: ICU length of stay, ICU acquired infections, hospital length of stay.

RESULTS

- At 28 days, there was a trend toward increased mortality among patients who received glutamine as compared with patients who did not receive glutamine (32.4% vs. 27.2%; p = 0.05).

- There was no significant difference in mortality between patients who receive antioxidant supplementation and patients who did not receive antioxidants (30.8% and 28.8%, respectively; $P = 0.48$).
- There was no significant interaction between glutamine and antioxidants ($P = 0.49$).
- No differences in 28-day mortality in a priori subgroup analyses.
- In-hospital and 6-month mortality were significantly higher among patients who received glutamine than among those who did not.
- Glutamine had no effect on the rates of organ failure or infectious complications.
- Antioxidants had no effect on 28-day mortality (30.8%, vs. 28.8% with no antioxidants; $P = 0.48$) or any other secondary end point (Table 35.1).

Table 35.1. SUMMARY OF REDOXS TRIAL KEY FINDINGS

Outcome	Glutamine	Antioxidants
28-day mortality	1.28 (1.00–1.64, p = 0.05)	1.09 (0.86–1.40, p = 0.48)

Criticisms and Limitations: The findings in this contrasted with the results of earlier studies which showed a potential benefit with glutamine supplementation in critically ill patients. However, these earlier studies were conducted in critically ill patients who did not have multi-organ failure. In particular, patients who were in shock were excluded from earlier studies. Additionally, in this study, unlike the previous ones, glutamine was administered via both parenteral and enteral administration, whereas prior studies used either parental or enteral formulation. The REDOXS trial also initiated earlier supplementation without adjunctive nutrition. The addition of glutamine that constituted 60% of total dietary protein introduced an amino acid imbalance with the potential for toxicity. Finally the rationale for early supplementation was based on the belief that critically ill patients were likely to be deficient in glutamine. However, measurements of glutamine levels performed in the study did not support this.

Other Relevant Studies and Information:

- Several reviews and meta-analyses have revisited the value of glutamine supplementation in critically-ill patients. The role of glutamine supplementation in critically ill patients remains a matter of open investigation.[2,3]
- Post hoc analysis of the REDOXS trial concluded that for both glutamine and antioxidants, the greatest potential for harm was

observed in patients with multiorgan failure that included renal dysfunction upon study enrollment.[4]

- Administering glutamine at a later time during the course of the patient's critical illness might have benefit.[3]

Summary and Implications: In the REDOXS trial, glutamine supplementation among critically ill patients was associated with increased mortality, an unexpected finding. Still, other research suggests a potential benefit of glutamine supplementation in the critically ill. The role of glutamine supplementation in critically ill patients remains a matter of open investigation.

CLINICAL CASE: EARLY SUPPLEMENTATION WITH GLUTAMINE IN CRITICALLY ILL PATIENTS

Case History:

A 65-year-old male admitted to the ICU after a Hartmann's procedure for diverticulitis and feculent peritonitis requiring mechanical ventilation support with a PaO_2/FiO_2 ratio of 200. Six hours into his admission, he clinically deteriorates with evidence of septic shock requiring increasing norepinephrine support and of ARDS and acute kidney injury.

Based on the results of the REDOXS trial, should glutamine supplementation be started early on this patient?

Suggested Answer:

The REDOXS trial showed that early supplementation in critically ill patients did not improve 28-day mortality rates and might increase mortality. However, supplementation with glutamine has been shown in other studies and reviews to be beneficial in those patients who are not in a shock state. Therefore, supplementation with glutamine may be considered once the patient is well resuscitated and without multi-organ failure.

References

1. Heyland D, et al., A randomized trial of glutamine and antioxidants in critically ill patients. *N Engl J Med.* 2013; 368(16): 1489–1497.
2. Mulherin DW, Sacks GS, Uncertainty about the safety of supplemental glutamine: an editorial on "A randomized trial of glutamine and antioxidants in critically ill patients." *Hepatobiliary Surg Nutr.* 2015; 4(1): 76–79.
3. Preiser JC, Wernerman J. REDOXs: important answers, many more questions raised! JPEN *J Parenter Enteral Nutr.* 2013; 37(5): 566–567.
4. Heyland DK, Elke G, Cook D, et al. Glutamine and antioxidants in the critically ill patient: a post hoc analysis of a large-scale randomized trial. *J Parenter Enteral Nutr.* 2015;39(4):401–409.

Renal

36

Low-Dose Dopamine in Patients with Early Renal Dysfunction

TAO SHEN

"Administration of low-dose dopamine by continuous intravenous infusion to critically ill patients at risk of renal failure does not confer clinically significant protection from renal dysfunction".
—BELLOMO ET AL.

Research Question: Does low-dose dopamine reduce the risk of renal failure in at-risk patients in the intensive care unit (ICU)?[1]

Sponsor: Australian and New Zealand Intensive Care Society (ANZICS) Clinical Trials Group

Year Study Began: 1996

Year Study Published: 2000

Study Location: 23 ICUs in Australia, New Zealand, and Hong Kong.

Who Was Studied: Patients aged over 18 years in the ICU with central venous catheters, who demonstrated ≥ 2 features of systemic inflammatory syndrome (SIRS) over a 24 hour period and at least one indicator of early renal dysfunction (urine output < 0.5 mL/kg hourly over ≥4 hours; serum creatinine concentration > 150 μmol/L in the absence of premorbid renal dysfunction; a rise in serum creatinine concentration of > 80 μmol/L within 24 hours in the absence of creatine kinase > 5000 IU/L or myoglobin in the urine).

Who Was Excluded: Patients who had acute renal failure within the previous 3 months, prior kidney transplant, use of dopamine during the current hospitalization, baseline serum creatinine concentration > 300 μmol/L, or those deemed unsuitable to receive dopamine or renal replacement therapy according to the enrolling physician.

How Many Patients: 467 patients were screened, 328 patients were enrolled; 4 were excluded from analysis

Study Overview: See Figure 36.1 for an overview of the study design.

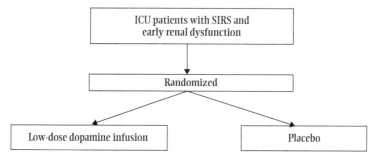

Figure 36.1 Summary of the study design.

Study Intervention: Patients admitted to the ICU were randomly assigned a continuous intravenous infusion of low-dose dopamine at 2 μg/kg/min or placebo through a central venous line. The infusions were continued until renal replacement therapy, death, discharge from ICU or resolution of SIRS and renal dysfunction for > 24 hours. All care providers and research personnel were blinded to the randomization process.

Follow-Up: To hospital discharge or death

Endpoints: The primary outcome was peak serum creatinine concentration reached during trial infusion. Secondary outcomes included urine output, need for renal replacement therapy, development of cardiac arrhythmias, duration of mechanical ventilation, duration of ICU and hospital stay, and survival to hospital discharge.

RESULTS

- Dopamine and placebo groups had similar baseline characteristics, renal function, and duration of infusion. The average length of infusion

was more than 4 days. Most study patients had septic shock and were receiving mechanical ventilation at the time of enrollment.
- There was no difference between the dopamine and placebo groups, respectively, in peak serum creatinine concentration (245 vs. 249 μmol; $p = 0.91$).
- There were no differences in secondary outcome measures, including changes in urine output, need for renal replacement therapy (21.7% with dopamine vs. 24.5% with placebo), duration of ICU or hospital stay, and survival to ICU and hospital discharge.
- When separately analyzing the subgroup of patients who stopped infusion due to resolution of renal dysfunction, no difference in time to renal recovery was found.
- Cardiac arrhythmias were equally common in both groups, with atrial fibrillation being the most common (Table 36.1).

Table 36.1. SUMMARY OF TRIAL RESULTS

	Dopamine ($n = 161$)	Placebo ($n = 163$)
Serum concentrations*	245 μmol/L	249 μmol/L
Peak creatinine	20 μmol/L	23 μmol/L
Peak urea		
Renal replacement therapy	35 patients (21.7%)	40 patients (24.5%)
Urine output*	37 mL/h	50 mL/h
Baseline	96 mL/h	92 mL/h
After 24 h	99 mL/h	109 mL/h
After 48 h		
Duration of mechanical ventilation*	10 days	11 days
Duration of ICU stay*	13 days	14 days
Duration of hospital stay*	29 days	33 days
Survival to ICU discharge	108 patients (67.1%)	105 patients (64.4%)
Cardiac arrhythmias	53 patients (32.9%)	54 (33.1%)

*Mean

Criticisms and Limitations:

- The study did not account for the administration of other drugs during the infusion period, which may affect urine output or glomerular filtration rate, such as diuretics and vasoactive drugs.
- The study population was heterogeneous including patients from a wide variety of medical and surgical ICUs, which may have diluted the benefits, if any, for a specific subgroup.

- Peak serum creatinine, the primary outcome measurement used in the study, can be affected by a number of factors, including age, muscle mass, and metabolism, which can in turn confound the interpretation of glomerular filtration rate and renal function in the study patients.
- The baseline mean central venous pressures and their standard deviations in table 1 of the study suggest that a subset of patients with low filling pressures were included in the study. It has been suggested that inadequate fluid resuscitation of this subset may account, at least partly, for the negative results
- The mean dose of furosemide was substantially less (192 mg) in the dopamine group compared with that in the placebo group (268 mg), which suggests differences in urine output between study groups that may have confounded the results.

Other Relevant Studies and Information:

- The rationale for the use of dopamine for preservation of renal function is based on findings in healthy humans and experimental animals showing that dopamine increases renal blood flow through dopamine-1 receptor mediated renal vasodilatation, which induces natriuresis and diuresis.[2,3]
- Several other clinical trials have also failed to show a benefit of low-dose dopamine on survival or the need for renal replacement therapy in critically ill patients.[4,5,6] In fact, the altered nature of drug metabolism, protein-binding and clearance in ICU patients challenges the very concept of selective renovascular low-dose dopamine infusion, as the effective serum concentration of dopamine may be highly variable in these patients, and any improved renal perfusion may reflect the systemic impact of beta-adrenergic effects on heart rate and cardiac output.
- Similarly, low-dose dopamine has not been proven to be beneficial in patients undergoing elective major vascular surgery,[7] coronary artery bypass grafting,[8] or liver and renal transplantation.[9,10]
- A meta-analysis of 61 trials and 3359 patients identified no benefit of low-dose dopamine on mortality, need for renal replacement therapy or adverse events, except that it was associated with a transient increase in urine output.[11]
- Low-dose dopamine is not without side effects. Dopamine can depress the respiratory drive, increase cardiac output and myocardial oxygen demand, induce hypokalemia and hypophosphatemia, predispose to gut ischemia, and cause metabolic and immunologic disruption by affecting a variety of hormones and T-cell function.[12,13] Of note, dopamine is

also a proximal tubular diuretic and by increasing the presentation and reabsorption of chloride ions in the ascending limb of the loop of Henle; consequently, dopamine may in fact increase medullary oxygen demand and exacerbate medullary ischemia.[1]

• For patients with established acute renal failure in the ICU, low-dose dopamine may actually worsen renal perfusion by increasing renal vascular resistance, although the mechanism of this is unclear.[14]

Summary and Implications: This study, along with several others, suggests that low-dose dopamine does not confer a clinically significant degree of renal protection in critically ill patients with SIRS who are at risk of renal failure. Given that dopamine is associated with a variety of adverse effects and that the drug's effect may be unpredictable in ICU patients, the administration of "renal-dose" dopamine in critically ill patients has fallen out of favor.

CLINICAL CASE: LOW-DOSE DOPAMINE IN PATIENTS WITH EARLY RENAL DYSFUNCTION

Case History:

A 78-year-old woman with coronary artery disease, hypertension, and type II diabetes is admitted to the ICU with community acquired pneumonia. She is tachycardic, hypotensive, and requiring supplemental oxygen via a facemask. Her urine output has dropped from 40–50 mL/hour to less than 10 mL/hour for the last several hours. Her serum creatinine is rising. Based on the results of this study, should the patient receive low-dose dopamine to prevent further deterioration of her renal function?

Suggested Answer:

This patient has severe pneumonia complicated by septic shock and most likely pre-renal acute renal dysfunction from systemic hypotension. According to the study, there is no benefit of using low-dose dopamine, as it makes no difference in this patient's risk of progressing to renal failure, need for dialysis, or overall survival. The metabolism and clearance of dopamine in this patient may also be unpredictable, which places her at increased risk for adverse effects of dopamine at higher serum concentrations, such as tachyarrhythmia, increased myocardial oxygen demand and decreased respiratory drive. The management of this patient centers on the timely administration of appropriate antibiotics, fluid resuscitation, and vasopressors, which help to correct sepsis-induced vasodilatation and renal perfusion.

References

1. Bellomo R, Chapman M, Finfer S, et al. Low-dose dopamine in patients with early renal dysfunction: a placebo-controlled randomized trial. Australian and New Zealand Intensive Care Society (ANZICS) Clinical Trials Group. *Lancet.* 2000; 356:2139–2143.
2. McDonald Jr R, Goldberg L, McNay J, Tuttle E. Effects of dopamine in man: augmentation of sodium excretion, glomerular filtration rate and renal plasma flow. *J Clin Invest.* 1964; 43:1116–1124.
3. Hollenberg N, Adams D, Mendall P, et al. Renal vascular responses to dopamine: hemodynamic and angiographic observations in normal man. *Clin Sci.* 1973; 45:733–742.
4. Marik P, Iglesias J. Low-dose dopamine does not prevent acute renal failure in patients with septic shock and oliguria. NORASEPT II Study Investigators. *Am J Med.* 1999; 107:392–395.
5. Flancbaum L, Choban P, Dasta J. Quantitative effects of low-dose dopamine on urine output in oliguric surgical intensive care unit patients. *Crit Care Med.* 1994; 22: 61–8.
6. Chertow G, Sayegh M, Allgren R, Lazarus J. Is the administration of dopamine associated with adverse or favorable outcomes in acute renal failure? Auriculin Anaritide Acute Renal Failure Study Group. *Am J Med.* 1999; 107:392–395.
7. Baldwin L, Henderson A, Hickman P. Effect of postoperative low-dose dopamine on renal function after elective major vascular surgery. *Ann Intern Med.* 1994; 120:744–747.
8. Myles PS, Buckland MR, Schenk NJ, et al. Effect of "renal-dose" dopamine on renal function following cardiac surgery. *Anaesth Intensive Care.* 1993; 21:56–61.
9. Swygert TH, Roberts LC, Valek TR, et al. Effect of intraoperative low-dose dopamine on renal function in liver transplant recipients. *Anesthesiology.* 1991; 75:571–576.
10. Kadieva V, Friedman L, Margolius L, Jackson SA, Morrell D. The effect of dopamine on graft function in patients undergoing renal transplantation. *Anesth Analges.* 1993; 76:362–365.
11. Friedrich J, Adhikari N, Herridge M, Beyene J. Meta-analysis: low-dose dopamine increases urine output but does not prevent renal dysfunction or death. *Ann Intern Med.* 2005; 142:510–524.
12. Denton M, Chertow G, Brady H. "Renal-dose" dopamine for the treatment of acute renal failure: scientific rationale, experimental studies and clinical trials. *Kidney Int.* 1996; 49:4–14.
13. Van den Berghe G, de Zegher F. Anterior pituitary function during critical illness and dopamine treatment. *Crit Care Med.* 1996; 24:1580–1590.
14. Lauschke A, Teichgraber U, Frei U, Eckardt K. 'Low-dose' dopamine worsens renal perfusion in patients with acute renal failure. *Kidney Int.* 2006; 69:1669–1674.

Intensity of Renal Support in Critically Ill Patients with Acute Kidney Injury

ERIC EHIELI AND YURIY BRONSHTEYN

"... a strategy of intensive renal support in critically ill patients with acute kidney injury does not decrease mortality, accelerate recovery of kidney function, or alter the rate of nonrenal organ failure as compared with a less-intensive regimen similar to usual-care practices."

—THE VA/NIH ACUTE RENAL FAILURE TRIAL NETWORK

Research Question: Do critically ill patients with severe acute kidney injury (AKI) benefit from a strategy of more-intensive renal replacement therapy (RRT) as compared with a strategy of less-intensive RRT?[1]

Year Study Began: 2003

Year Study Published: 2008

Study Location: 27 VA and university-affiliated medical centers

Who Was Studied: Adults with AKI clinically consistent with acute tubular necrosis (ATN) defined by an ischemic or nephrotoxic injury and oliguria for >1 day or a rise in serum creatinine or ≥2 mg/dL in males of ≥1.5 mg/dl in females over a period of < 4 days, as well as failure of one or more non-renal organ systems as defined by non-renal Sepsis Organ Failure Assessment (SOFA) ≥2 (with a higher score indicating more severe organ dysfunction or sepsis).

Who Was Excluded: Patients with: baseline serum creatinine > 2 mg/dL
(> 1.5 mg/dL in females); AKI clinically believed to be from an etiology other
than ATN, or deemed not a candidate for RRT due to futility (e.g., terminal condition); > 72 hours since fulfilling the definition of ARF and BUN > 100 mg/dL ;
> 1 session of intermittent hemodialysis or sustained low-efficiency dialysis or
more than 24 hours of continuous renal-replacement therapy before randomization; prior kidney transplant; pregnancy; prisoner; weight > 128.5 kg.

How Many Patients: 1124

Study Overview: See Figure 37.1 for a summary of the study design.

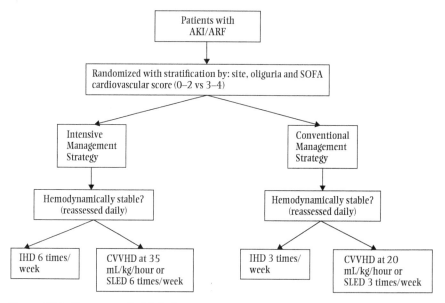

Figure 37.1 Summary of trial design.

Study Intervention: In both the intensive and conventional management
groups, patients underwent IHD when they were hemodynamically stable
(defined as having a SOFA cardiovascular score ≤ 2) and underwent CVVHD
or sustained low-efficiency dialysis (SLED) when they were hemodynamically
unstable (SOFA cardiovascular score of 3 to 4). The selection of CVVHD or SLED
was determined by site-specific practice. Patients were transitioned from IHD to
CVVHD or SLED if they became hemodynamically unstable and from CVVHD
or SLED to IHD when hemodynamic instability resolved (for > 24 hours).

In the group receiving the intensive RRT, IHD or SLED were provided 6
times per week, and CVVHD was prescribed to provide a flow rate of the total
effluent (the sum of the dialysate and ultrafiltrate) of 35 mL/kg/hour. In the

less-intensive RRT group, IDH and SLED were provided three times per week, and CVVHD was prescribed to provide a total effluent flow rate of 20 mL per kilogram per hour. In both treatment groups, intermittent hemodialysis and sustained low-efficiency hemodialysis were prescribed to provide a single-pool Kt/V_{urea} (an index of the dialysis dose in which K is the urea clearance of the dialyzer, t is the duration of dialysis, and V is the volume of distribution of urea) of 1.2 to 1.4 per session.

The assigned renal-replacement therapy was provided for up to 28 days after randomization or until recovery of kidney function, discharge from acute care, withdrawal of life-sustaining therapy, or death. . In patients with persistent renal failure 28 days after randomization, or in those who were discharged from acute care before day 28, further RRT was at the discretion of the treating clinicians.

Follow-Up: 60 days

Endpoints: Primary outcome: All-cause mortality by day 60. Secondary outcomes: Duration of RRT, in-hospital mortality by day 60, renal recovery by day 60 (complete or partial), intensive care unit (ICU) and hospital length of stay, days of non-renal organ dysfunction, and whether patient returned home and did not require dialysis by day 60.

RESULTS

- There was no significant difference between the two groups with regard to in-hospital or 60-day mortality (53.6% in the intensive-therapy group vs 51.5% undergoing less-intensive; $P = 0.47$).
- There was no significant difference between the two groups with regard to recovery of kidney function by day 28 (15.4% of all patients in the intensive-therapy group had complete recovery of kidney function and 8.9% had partial recovery, as compared with 18.4% and 9.0%, respectively, receiving less-intensive therapy; $P = 0.24$).
- There was no significant difference between the two groups in the incidence of successful discharge home off dialysis by day 60 (15.7% undergoing intensive therapy as compared with 16.4%) undergoing less-intensive therapy ($P = 0.75$).
- There was no significant difference between the groups with regard to hospital-free and ICU-free days through day 60.
- The intensive RRT group experienced significantly higher rates of hypotension requiring vasopressor support (14.4 vs. 10%; $P = 0.02$), hypophosphatemia (17.6% vs. 10.9%; $P = 0.001$), and hypokalemia (7.5% vs. 4.5%; $P = 0.03$) (Table 37.1).

Table 37.1. SUMMARY OF KEY FINDINGS

Outcome	Intensive RRT	Less Intensive RRT	P Value
All-cause mortality by day 60	53.6%	51.5%	0.47
In-hospital mortality	51.2%	48.0%	0.27
Home by day 60 with complete renal recovery	15.7%	16.4%	0.75
Hypotension requiring vasopressor support	14.4%	10.0%	0.02
Hypophosphatemia	17.6%	10.9%	0.001
Hypokalemia	7.5%	4.5%	0.03

Criticisms and Limitations: Men are overrepresented in this study population (VA patients comprised 25% of the study patients), thus raising the question of the extent to which its results can be generalized to female patients.

The study excluded patients with advanced chronic kidney disease and therefore the findings may not be generalizable to a large number of ICU patients with CKD who develop AKI requiring RRT.

Other Relevant Studies and Information:

- Prior to this study, a number of smaller studied showed improved outcomes with intensive RRT,[2–4] whereas others showed no improved benefit from intensive RRT.[5,6]
- The results of this study were replicated by another similar RCT that compared lower intensity continuous RRT (25 mL/kg/hour effluent flow) versus higher intensity (40 mL/kg/hour) in critically ill patients. The authors found no difference in either death or need for RRT at 28 days and 90 days of follow-up.[7]
- More recent studies have shown that while persistently elevated inflammatory biomarkers are associated with RRT dependence and death,[8,9] it is unclear whether reducing these markers with early intensive RRT is associated with better outcomes.[10]
- A Cochrane systematic review and meta-analysis six studies comparing intensive and less intensive CRRT did not demonstrate beneficial effects on mortality or recovery of kidney function in critically ill patients with AKI.[11]
- KDIGO practice guidelines from recommend a less intensive RRT regimen (delivering an effluent volume of 20–25 mL/kg/h for CRRT in AKI and delivering a Kt/V of 3.9 per week when using intermittent or extended RRT in AKI.[12]

Summary and Implications: In critically ill patients with severe AKI from ATN, a strategy of intensive RRT does not appear to improve survival, improve renal recovery, or alter the rate of non-renal organ failure, as compared with less intensive RRT practice. Moreover, more intensive RRT was associated with more hypotension requiring vasopressor support, hypokalemia, and hypophosphatemia.

CLINICAL CASE: LOW- VERSUS HIGH-INTENSITY RENAL REPLACEMENT THERAPY IN THE ICU

Case History:

A 75-year-old male was admitted to the intensive care unit with septic shock from staphylococcal aureus bacteremia and endocarditis. He had normal kidney function prior to admission but developed acute kidney injury. His urine sediment reveals muddy brown granular casts. He remains in the intensive care unit and now requires initiation of renal replacement therapy (RRT). What is the ideal intensity of RRT for this patient: 20 mL/kg versus 35 mL/kg of effluent flow?

Suggested Answer:

The study by Ronco et al. showed that low-intensity RRT was non-inferior to high-intensity RRT for patients with acute kidney injury requiring renal replacement therapy. Patients treated with low-intensity RRT had the same rates of in-hospital and 60-day mortality but low rates of hypotension and electrolyte deficiency compared to patients that received high-intensity RRT.

This patient was typical of the patients included in the trial by Ronco et al: a patient with previously normal kidney function who developed new-onset acute kidney injury in the hospital. For patients receiving intermittent hemodialysis (IHD, the study showed similar results when comparing low-intensity (IHD 3 times/week) versus high-intensity (IHD 6 times/week).

References

1. VA/NIH Acute Renal Failure Trial Network. Intensity of renal support in critically ill patients with acute kidney injury. *New Engl J Med.* 2008;359(1):7–20.
2. Ronco C, Bellomo R, Homel P, et al. Effects of different doses in continuous venovenous haemofiltration on outcomes of acute renal failure: a prospective randomised trial. *Lancet.* 2000;356(9223):26–30.

3. Saudan P, Niederberger M, De Seigneux S, et al. Adding a dialysis dose to continuous hemofiltration increases survival in patients with acute renal failure. *Kidney Int.* 2006;70(7):1312–1317.
4. Schiffl H, Lang SM, Fischer R. Daily hemodialysis and the outcome of acute renal failure. *New Engl J Med.* 2002;346(5):305–310.
5. Tolwani AJ, Campbell RC, Stofan BS, Lai KR, Oster RA, Wille KM. Standard versus high-dose CVVHDF for ICU-related acute renal failure. *J Am Soc Nephrol.* 2008;19(6):1233–1238.
6. Bouman CS, Oudemans-Van Straaten HM, Tijssen JG, Zandstra DF, Kesecioglu J. Effects of early high-volume continuous venovenous hemofiltration on survival and recovery of renal function in intensive care patients with acute renal failure: a prospective, randomized trial. *Crit Care Med.* 2002;30(10):2205–2211.
7. RENAL Replacement Therapy Study Investigators, Bellomo R, Cass A, Cole L. et al Intensity of continuous renal-replacement therapy in critically ill patients. *New Engl J Med.* 2009;361(17):1627–1638.
8. Payen D, Lukaszewicz AC, Legrand M, et al. A multicentre study of acute kidney injury in severe sepsis and septic shock: association with inflammatory phenotype and HLA genotype. *PloS One.* 2012;7(6):e35838.
9. Murugan R, Wen X, Shah N, et al. Plasma inflammatory and apoptosis markers are associated with dialysis dependence and death among critically ill patients receiving renal replacement therapy. *Nephrology, dialysis, transplantation: Official Publication of the European Dialysis and Transplant Association—European Renal Association.* 2014;29(10):1854–1864.
10. Ronco C, Ricci Z, De Backer D, et al. Renal replacement therapy in acute kidney injury: controversy and consensus. *Critical Care.* 2015;19:146.
11. Fayad AI, Buamscha DG, Ciapponi A. Intensity of continuous renal replacement therapy for acute kidney injury. *Cochrane Database Syst Rev.* 2016;10:CD010613.
12. Khwaja A. KDIGO clinical practice guidelines for acute kidney injury. *Nephron Clin Pract.* 2012;120(4):c179–184.

38

Continuous Venovenous Hemodiafiltration versus Intermittent Hemodialysis for Acute Renal Failure in Patients with Multiple-Organ Dysfunction Syndrome

A Multicenter Randomized Trial

CHRISTINA ANNE JELLY AND EDWARD BITTNER

"60-day survival rates for acute renal failure in multiple-organ-dysfunction syndrome do not differ when continuous renal replacement therapy or intermittent haemodialysis are used."

—VINSONNEAU ET AL.

Research Question: Does continuous renal replacement therapy (CRRT) have a survival benefit compared with intermittent hemodialysis (IHD) for the treatment of acute renal failure in critically ill patients?[1]

Sponsor: Société de Réanimation de Langue Française

Year Study Began: 1999

Year Study Published: 2006

Study Location: 21 medical or multidisciplinary intensive-care units in university or community hospitals in France

Who Was Studied: Patients with acute renal failure requiring renal replacement therapy as part of multiple-organ dysfunction syndrome. Acute renal failure was defined as one of the following (1) serum urea concentration greater than 36 mmol/L ; (2)serum creatinine more than 310 umol/L; or (3) oliguria defined as a urine output of less than 320 mL for 16 hours, despite appropriate fluid loading. Presence of multiple-organ dysfunction syndrome was defined by a logistic organ dysfunction score of 6 or more.

Who Was Excluded: Patients who were pregnant, younger than 18 years of age, preexisting chronic renal failure, acute renal failure of obstructive or vascular origin, ongoing treatment with an ACE inhibitor, coagulation disorders, uncontrolled hemorrhage, moribund state or those with a survival expectancy of fewer than 8 days.

How Many Patients: 360

Study Overview: See Figure 38.1 for an overview of the study design.

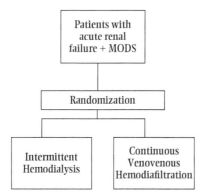

Figure 38.1 Summary of trial design.

Study Intervention: Patients were randomized to receive either continuous renal replacement therapy ($n = 176$) or intermittent hemodialysis ($n = 184$). Investigators were provided with recommendations on how to achieve optimum metabolic control and hemodynamic stability during the intervention. For CRRT, the recommendations included an initial blood flow of 120 mL/minute or more, dialysate flow of 500 mL/hour or more, and ultrafiltration flow of 1000 mL/hour or more. For IHD, the recommendations included initial blood flow of 250 mL/minute or more and dialysate flow set at 500 mL/minute. The two groups were treated with the same polymer membrane and bicarbonate-based buffer. All investigators started the randomized therapy with initial standardized settings and then adapted the settings to meet individual patient needs for optimal metabolic control.

Optimum metabolic control was defined as maintaining a urea concentration of less than 30 mmol/L in the CRRT group and as a urea reduction ratio greater than 65% per session for the IHD group.

Follow-Up: 90 days

Endpoints: Primary outcome: 60-day survival. Secondary outcomes: 28-day and 90-day survival, length of stay in intensive care and in hospital, duration of extra-renal support, recovery of renal function, and occurrence of adverse events.

RESULTS

- There was no significant difference in the mean 60-day survival between the IHD (31.5%) and CRRT (32.6%) groups. Survival was also similar between groups at all other times throughout the study. However, there was a progressive and significant increase in the survival rate in the IHD group over time, while the survival was constant over time in the CRRT group.
- There were no differences in the length of stay in the intensive care unit or in the hospital between the two groups.
- There were no differences in the rate and time to recovery of renal function between the two groups.
- The incidence of adverse events, such as hypotension and thrombocytopenia, did not differ significantly throughout the course of the study between groups (Table 38.1).

Table 38.1. SUMMARY OF THE STUDY'S KEY FINDINGS

Outcome	IHD	CVVHDF	P value
60-day survival	31.5%	32.6%	0.98
Renal support duration (days)	11	11	0.84
Length of ICU stay (days)	20	19	0.73
Length of hospital stay (days)	30	32	0.66

Criticisms and Limitations:

- Despite being among the largest randomized controlled trial to date comparing CRRT to IHD the study may have been underpowered. The study was designed to detect a 15% absolute difference in mortality with a sample size of 240 patients in each group, which was not achieved.
- The study did not comprehensively compare the delivered dialysis dose between treatment groups which has been shown to influence mortality in some studies. The study by Vinsonneau et al reported that the

mean dialysis dose was only 29 mL/kg/hour among the CRRT group; however, the delivered dose in IHD group was not available to compare.

- The finding that the mortality rate in the IHD group decreased significantly overtime, whereas mortality in the CRRT group remained stable is unexplained. The authors raised the possibility that standard of care improvements during the study could have favored IHD, but found no evidence of such an effect is provided.

Other Relevant Studies and Information:

- Several theoretical advantages have been attributed to CRRT over IHD in critically ill patients including more hemodynamic stability allowing more adequate fluid removal, better recovery of renal function, and more efficient removal of small and large metabolites. Some supporters of CRRT also suggest the benefit of enhanced cytokine removal, but the clinical significance of this theoretical advantage remains unknown.
- Recent meta-analyses have failed to consistently demonstrate a better hemodynamic stability and/or superior vital parameters for CRRT, a difference in dialysis dependence or general survival benefit for either RRT strategy.[2,3,4]
- The recently published "CONVINT" trial randomized critically ill patients with dialysis-dependent acute renal failure to receive either daily IHD or CVVHDF. Furthermore no differences were observed in mortality, days on RRT, vasopressor days, days on ventilator, or ICU/hospital length of stay, thus adding further support that IHD and CRRTs may be considered equivalent approaches for critically ill patients with dialysis-dependent acute renal failure.[5]
- IHD has been suspected to cause long-term chronic kidney disease in previously critically ill acute kidney injury patients. If this suspicion is confirmed, IHD as a first-line treatment in the ICU should be reserved for patients who are less likely to be weaned from RRT.
- The question of which RRT is better may be determined by the nature of the task. CRRT may be better in terms of hemodynamic stability and total water and solute removal over 24 hours awhile IHD can remove much more water and solute per hour, is not associated with the need for continuous anticoagulation, and does not require continuous patient immobilization.
- The KDIGO (Kidney Disease: Improving Global Outcomes) clinical practice guideline for acute kidney injury (AKI) recommends using CRRT, rather than standard intermittent RRT, for hemodynamically unstable patients and for patients with acute brain injury, other causes of increased intracranial pressure or generalized brain edema.[6]

Summary and Implications: This study, suggests that critically ill patients with acute renal failure and multiple organ dysfunction can be treated with intermittent hemodialysis if appropriate attention is paid to hemodynamic and metabolic control. Although CRRT may be a more convenient method for renal replacement therapy in critically ill patients, its potential advantage must be weighed against its substantially higher cost and the lack of proven added clinical benefit.

CLINICAL CASE: CONTINUOUS VENOVENOUS HEMODIAFILTRATION VERSUS INTERMITTENT HEMODIALYSIS

Case History:

A 72-year-old male with past medical history of hypertension, diabetes, chronic renal insufficiency (baseline creatinine of 2.2 mg/dL), and recurrent small bowel obstructions admitted to the intensive care unit after an emergent exploratory laparotomy for a closed loop small bowel obstruction. The patient was oliguric in the operating room and in the ICU has not made any urine in 6 hours. His most recent laboratory panel is notable for a potassium level of 6.5 mEq/L. He remains intubated and sedated and has required 20–40 mcg/minute of phenylephrine for blood pressure support. The consulting renal physician recommends intermittent hemodialysis. How do you respond?

Suggested Answer:

Renal replacement therapy is indicated for this critically ill patient with hyperkalemia and oliguria. Either IHD or continuous venovenous hemodiafiltration (CVVHDF) would be appropriate as the existing data has not shown any difference in mortality among the two modalities in critically ill patients. Intermittent hemodialysis would offer several advantages such as more rapid clearance of acidosis, uremia, and electrolytes while removing less amino acids, endogenous hormones, and cofactors. IHD also results in less hypothermia and greater patient mobility and would not require anticoagulation. However, the major advantage of CVVHDF in this patient would be greater hemodynamic stability, especially in the setting of ongoing vasopressor use.

References

1. Vinsonneau C, Camus C, Combes A, et al. Continuous venovenous haemodiafiltration versus intermittent haemodialysis for acute renal failure in patients with multiple-organ dysfunction syndrome: a multicentre randomised trial. *Lancet.* 2006; 368:379–385.

2. Friedrich JO, Wald R, Bagshaw SM, Burns KE, Adhikari NKJ. Hemofiltration compared to hemodialysis for acute kidney injury: systematic review and meta-analysis. *Crit Care.* 2012;16:R146.
3. Bagshaw SM, Berthiaume LR, Delaney A, Bellomo R. Continuous versus intermittent renal replacement therapy for critically ill patients with acute kidney injury: a meta-analysis. *Crit Care Med.* 2008;36:610–617.
4. Ghahramani N, Shadrou S, Hollenbeak C. A systematic review of continuous renal replacement therapy and intermittent haemodialysis in management of patients with acute renal failure. *Nephrology (Carlton)* 2008;13:570–578.
5. Schefold JC, von Haehling S, Pschowski R, et al. The effect of continuous versus intermittent renal replacement therapy on the outcome of critically ill patients with acute renal failure (CONVINT): a prospective randomized controlled trial. *Crit Care.* 2014;18(1):R11.
6. http://www.kdigo.org/clinical_practice_guidelines/pdf/KDIGO%20AKI%20 Guideline.pdf. Last accessed 3/22/2017.

Hematologic

39

A Multicenter, Randomized, Controlled Clinical Trial of Transfusion Requirements in Critical Care

The Transfusion Requirements in Critical Care (TRICC) Trial

JOSEPH R. GUENZER AND ANDREW VARDANIAN

"A restrictive strategy of red-cell transfusion is at least as effective as and possibly superior to a liberal transfusion strategy in critically ill patients, with the possible exception of patients with acute myocardial infarction and unstable angina."

—HEBERT ET AL.

Research Question: Is a restrictive strategy of red-cell transfusion equivalent to a liberal transfusion strategy in critically ill patients?[1]

Year Study Began: 1994

Year Study Published: 1999

Study Location: Intensive care units (ICUs) in 22 tertiary hospitals and 3 community hospitals in Canada

Study Overview: See Figure 39.1 for an overview of the study design.

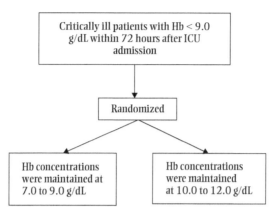

Figure 39.1 Summary of the study design.

Who Was Studied: Critically ill patients with a hemoglobin concentration of less than 9 g per deciliter (g/dL) within 72 hours after ICU admission who were expected to stay in the ICU for more than 24 hours and were deemed to be euvolemic by the attending physician after initial treatment.

Who Was Excluded: Patients who were under the age of 16, were unable to receive blood products, were experiencing ongoing blood loss at the time of enrollment, had chronic anemia, were pregnant, were brain dead or at risk of imminent death, or were admitted after a routine cardiac surgical procedure. Also excluded were patients whose treatment team was considering withholding or withdrawing ongoing treatment.

How Many Patients: 838 patients underwent randomization. The authors initially calculated they would need to enroll 2300 patients to detect a mortality difference of 4% assuming 18% mortality in the overall sample. This was later decreased to 1620 patients after an interim analysis showed the overall mortality to be 23%. However, enrollment was stopped early due to a decrease in enrollment to less than 20% of predicted levels. The low rate of consent was not explained by the authors.

Study Intervention: Patients were randomized to either a restrictive transfusion strategy where hemoglobin was maintained between 7.0 and 9.0 g per deciliter or a liberal transfusion strategy where the hemoglobin was maintained between 10.0 and 12.0 g per deciliter (Figure 39.1). Patients were transfused one unit of packed red blood cells (PRBCs) at a time if their hemoglobin concentration dropped below the lower limit of the target range. Hemoglobin concentrations were checked after each transfusion and transfusion was repeated until the value reached the goal range. The intervention strategy was maintained for the duration of the patient's ICU stay and was terminated at discharge from the ICU. All other care was at the discretion of the treating team.

Follow-Up: 60 days

Endpoints: Primary outcome was 30-day mortality. Secondary outcomes included 60-day mortality, in-ICU and in-hospital mortality, survival-times during the first 30 days, multiple-organ failure (MOF) scores, and multiple-organ dysfunction (MOD) scores. Pre-specified subgroup analyses were to be performed stratifying patients by age (older than 55, younger than 55), APACHE II score (greater than 20, less than 20), and presence of cardiac disease. A post hoc analysis was performed in patients with systemic infection.

RESULTS

- The average hemoglobin after randomization in the restrictive group was 8.5 +/−0.7 g/dL versus 10.7 +/− 0.7 g/dL in the liberal group. The liberal group was transfused significantly more often on a per patient basis. Adherence to protocol was greater than 98%.[1]
- There was a trend towards reduced mortality in the restrictive group (18.7% vs. 23.3% at 30 days) though this was not statistically significant ($p = 0.11$). This trend persisted to 60 days (22.7% vs. 26.5%, $p = 0.23$).
- There was no difference in unadjusted MOD scores. There was a statistically significant decrease in MOD scores in the restrictive group when adjusted to include patients who died within 30 days and assigning them the maximum scores.
- There was no difference in ICU (11.0 vs. 11.5 days, $p = 0.53$) or hospital (34.8 vs. 35.5 days, $p = 0.58$) length of stay.
- In pre-specified subgroup analyses, there was a statistically significant improvement in mortality in the restrictive group among patients less 55 years old (5.7% vs. 13.0%, $p = 0.02$) and with APACHE II score of 20 or less (8.7% vs. 16.1%, $p = 0.03$).
- There was no difference in mortality among patients with cardiac disease (20.5% vs. 22.9%, p = 0.69), septic shock (22.8% vs. 29.7%, $p = 0.36$), or trauma (10.0% vs. 8.8%, $p = 0.81$).
- There were statistically significant differences in cardiac complications, myocardial infarction, and pulmonary edema, though not acute respiratory distress syndrome (ARDS) between the 2 groups (Figure 39.2).

Criticisms and Limitations:

- The trial stopped enrollment early and as such was underpowered to prove equivalency. It is possible that complete enrollment would have shown that the restrictive strategy was associated with a decrease in mortality.
- The high rate of patient or provider refusal to consent may have skewed the study population toward a younger, healthier population, thereby limiting the generalizability of the study.
- It is possible that the low rate of enrollment preferentially excluded patients who were more likely to benefit from or be harmed by blood transfusion, thus leading to therapeutic misalignment. Specifically, the trial excludes cardiac surgical patients who make up a large proportion of the general ICU population.[2]
- The study was performed using non-leukocyte-reduced blood products. These products have now become the standard transfusion product at many large centers and throughout Australia and Canada and may be associated with a lower risk of potentially harmful complications.[3]

Other Relevant Studies:

- A randomized, controlled study of 998 patients admitted to the ICU with septic shock showed no difference in 90-day mortality between patients randomized to restrictive and liberal transfusion strategies (transfusion thresholds of < 7 g/dL and < 9 g/dL respectively) when using leukocyte-depleted PRBCs.[4]
- A randomized, controlled trial of 921 patients with severe, acute upper gastrointestinal bleeding showed improved mortality in the group randomized a restrictive transfusion strategy (transfusion threshold of < 7 g/dL) as opposed to a liberal strategy (transfusion threshold of < 9 g/dL).[5]
- In a study of high-risk patients who were anemic after hip surgery, no difference in mortality or ability to ambulate at 30 days was seen between restrictive and liberal transfusion strategies (transfusion thresholds of < 7 g/dL and < 9 g/dL respectively).[6]
- In the TRACS trial, post-cardiac surgery patients were randomized to either a restrictive (transfusion threshold hematocrit < 24%) or liberal (threshold hematocrit < 30%) transfusion strategy. No difference in a composite of 30-day mortality and severe morbidity was observed.[7]

Summary and Implications: The TRICC trial was the first large trial to examine the impact of transfusion thresholds on mortality in critically ill patients.

Though the trial was underpowered, the trend toward decreased mortality in the restrictive group does suggest that it is unlikely that the lower transfusion threshold subjects patients to increased harm. However, care must be taken in generalizing these results to cardiac surgery patients or to patients that are actively bleeding based on this study alone. Additionally, the increasingly common use of pre-storage leukocyte-reduction of PRBCs may diminish the harm of associated with increased transfusion.

CLINICAL CASE: USING THE TRICC TRIAL

Case History:
A 53-year-old man with acute myeloblastic leukemia who is hospitalized for induction chemotherapy is found to have new-onset altered mental status and hypoxemia and is found to have a new right lower lobe consolidation on chest radiograph. He is intubated for hypoxemia respiratory failure and transferred to the intensive care unit. Broad-spectrum antibiotics are initiated. The patient is neutropenic and has a hemoglobin concentration is 10.3 g/dL at presentation to the ICU. After fluid resuscitation with balanced salt solution, the hemoglobin drops to 7.8 g/dL. The patient is now oxygenating well and is hemodynamically stable. There is minimal respiratory variation on the arterial line waveform. Stool and nasogastric-tube output are non-bloody. Serum iron, ferritin, and transferrin saturation indicate that the patient is not iron-deficient. Should this patient be transfused for worsening anemia?

Suggested Answer:
The TRICC trial suggests that there is no increased harm from adhering to a more restrictive blood transfusion strategy where the hemoglobin concentration is maintained in the range of 7.0–10.0 g/dL and a transfusion threshold of 7.0 g/dL is used. In fact, this strategy may be superior to maintaining the hemoglobin at 10.0–12.0 g/dL with a transfusion threshold of 10.0 g/dL. Because this patient is not hypovolemic, is hemodynamically stable, is not actively bleeding, and is not recovering from cardiac surgery, he is typical of the patients enrolled in the TRICC trial.

References
1. Hebert PC, Wells G, Tweeddale M, et al. Transfusion Requirements in Critical Care (TRICC) Investigators and the Canadian Critical Care Trials Group. Does transfusion practice affect mortality in critically ill patients? *Am J Respir Crit Care Med.* 1997;155(5):1618–1623.

2. Cserti-Gazdewich CM. Hitting the tipping point of TRICC? *Transfusion.* 2010;50(10):2076–2079.

3. Hebert PC, Fergusson D, Blajchman MA, et al. Leukoreduction Study Investigators. Clinical outcomes following institution of the Canadian universal leukoreduction program for red blood cell transfusion. *JAMA.* 2003;289(15):1941–1949.

4. Holst LB, Haase N, Wetterslev J, et al. TRISS Trial Group; Scandinavian Critical Care Trials Group. Lower versus higher hemoglobin threshold for transfusion in septic shock. *N Engl J Med.* 2014;371(15):1381–1391.

5. Villanueva C, Colomo A, Bosch A, et al. Transfusion strategies for acute upper gastro-intestinal bleeding. *N Engl J Med.* 2013;368(1):11–21.

6. Carson KL, Terrin ML, Noveck H, et al. FOCUS Investigators. Liberal or restrictive transfusion in high-risk patients after hip surgery. *N Engl J Med.* 2011;365(26):2453–2462.

7. Hajjar LA, Vincent JL, Galas FR, et al. Transfusion requirements after cardiac surgery: the TRACS randomized controlled trial. *JAMA.* 2010;304(14):1559–1567.

40

Reducing Mortality Among Bleeding Trauma Patients with Tranexamic Acid

The CRASH-2 (Clinical Randomization of an Antifibrinolytic in Significant Hemorrhage-2) Randomized Controlled Trial

HAYTHAM M. A. KAAFARANI

"[E]arly administration of tranexamic acid to trauma patients with, or at risk for, significant bleeding reduces the risk of death from haemorrhage with no apparent increase in fatal or non-fatal vascular occlusive events."
—CRASH-2 TRIAL COLLABORATORS

Research Question: Can the administration of tranexamic acid, an anti-fibrinolytic agent, decrease the mortality of bleeding trauma patients?[1]

Sponsor: Funding was provided by the UK NIHR Health Technology Assessment Programme, Pfizer, BUPA Foundation, and J P Moulton Charitable Foundation

Year Study Began: 2005

Study Location: 274 hospitals in 40 countries

Who Was Studied: Adult trauma patients with significant bleeding within 8 h from injury and with a systolic blood pressure less than 90 mm Hg or heart rate more than 110 beats per minute were included. To be included, the treating physician needed to be "uncertain" on whether tranexamic acid was indicated.

Who Was Excluded: Patients in whom the treating physician felt there was either a clear indication or a clear contra-indication to the use of tranexamic acid were excluded. Four patients withdrew their consent after randomization and were not included in the intent-to-treat analysis.

How Many Patients: A total of 20,211 patients were randomized to receive either tranexamic acid or placebo.

Study Overview: In 274 hospitals from 40 countries, adult trauma patients presenting within 8 h from injury in hemorrhagic shock or deemed to be at risk for significant bleeding were randomized to receive either tranexamic acid or placebo (Figure 40.1).

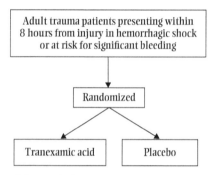

Figure 40.1 Summary of the study design.

Study Intervention: Once patients were deemed eligible, consent was obtained from them directly when possible, or from their proxy. If neither was feasible, consent was waived if allowed by local regulation. Randomization was then performed using a computer random number generator and an algorithm that balanced for center, country, age, gender, time since injury, type of injury, and presenting vital signs and neurological status. Patients received either a loading dose = 1 g followed by a 1 g infusion over 8 h, or its matching placebo. The tranexamic acid and placebo were contained in indistinguishable ampules. The patients, study staff and treatment teams were blinded to the treatment.

Follow-Up: Until patient discharge or 4 weeks post-injury

Endpoints: The primary outcome of the study was death in the hospital within 4 weeks of injury. The cause of death was also recorded (e.g., bleeding, myocardial infarction, stroke, pulmonary embolism, head injury, multi-organ failure). Secondary outcomes included vascular occlusive events (e.g., myocardial infarction, stroke, pulmonary embolism), the need for transfusion, the number of units of blood products received, and functional dependency (dead, fully or partially dependent vs. independent). All analyses were performed on an intention-to-treat basis.

RESULTS

- The two treatment groups were similar in terms of baseline characteristics (Table 40.1). Specifically, tranexamic acid and placebo patients were balanced in terms of age, gender, presenting time since injury, type of injury (blunt versus penetrating), presenting systolic blood pressure, presenting respiratory rate, presenting capillary refill time, presenting heart rate and presenting Glasgow Coma Scale.

Table 40.1. PATIENT RANDOMIZATION INTO TRANEXAMIC ACID
VERSUS PLACEBO

20,211 Patients Randomized

10,096 allocated to tranexamic acid	10,115 allocated to placebo
3 withdrew consent	1 withdrew consent
33 with no follow-up	47 with no follow-up
10,060 analyzed	10,067 analyzed

- A total of 3,076 patients died (15.3%), 35.3% of which died on the day of randomization.
- All-cause mortality was reduced from 16.0% in placebo patients to 14.5% in tranexamic acid patients (Table 40.2), $p = 0.0035$.

Table 40.2. MORTALITY AND CAUSES OF MORTALITY IN TRANEXAMIC ACID
VERSUS PLACEBO PATIENTS

Patient Group Cause of Death	Tranexamic acid ($N = 10060$), %	Placebo ($N = 10067$), %	Relative Risk (95% CI)	P Value
Any	1463 (14.5%)	1613 (16.0%)	0.91 (0.85–0.97)	0.0035
Bleeding	489 (4.9%)	574 (5.7%)	0.85 (0.76–0.96)	0.0077
Vascular occlusion	33 (0.3%)	48 (0.5%)	0.69 (0.44–1.07)	0.096
Multi-organ failure	209 (2.1%)	233 (2.3%)	0.90 (0.75–1.08)	0.25
Head injury	603 (6.0%)	621 (6.2%)	0.97 (0.87–1.08)	0.60
Other	129 (1.3%)	137 (1.4%)	0.94 (0.74–1.20)	0.63

Vascular Occlusion = myocardial infarction, stroke, pulmonary embolism

- Similarly, the risk of mortality from bleeding was reduced from 5.7% in placebo patients to 4.9% in tranexamic acid patients (Table 40.2), $p = 0.0077$. Mortality from other causes (e.g. vascular occlusion) was similar between the two groups.
- The rate of occurrence of vascular occlusive events (fatal or non-fatal), a potential side-effect of an antifibrinolytic agent like tranexamic acid, was similar between the two groups (1.7% vs. 2.0%, $p = 0.084$);

the rate of myocardial infarction was *lower* in the tranexamic acid
patients compared to the placebo patients (0.3% vs. 0.5%, respectively;
$p = 0.035$) (Table 40.3).

Table 40.3. TOTAL (FATAL AND NONFATAL) VASCULAR OCCLUSIVE EVENTS
AND BLOOD PRODUCTS TRANSFUSED

	Tranexamic acid ($N = 10060$), %	Placebo ($N = 10067$), %	Relative Risk (95% CI)	P Value
Myocardial Infarction	35 (0.3%)	55 (0.5%)	0.64 (0.42–0.97)	0.035
Stroke	57 (0.6%)	66 (0.7%)	0.86 (0.61–1.23)	0.42
Pulmonary embolism	72 (0.7%)	71 (0.7%)	1.01 (0.73–1.41)	0.93
Deep vein thrombosis	40 (0.4%)	41 (0.4%)	0.98 (0.63–1.51)	0.91
Blood product transfused	5067 (50.4%)	5160 (51.3%)	0.98 (0.96–1.01)	0.21

- The percentage of patients receiving blood products was similar
  between the tranexamic acid and the placebo groups (50.4% vs. 51.3%,
  respectively; $p = 0.21$)
- In pre-specified subgroup analyses (Figure 40.1), the tranexamic acid
  decreased mortality specifically among patients who presented less than
  3 h following their injury, and in patients with a systolic blood pressure
  less than or equal to 75 mm Hg.

Criticisms and Limitations:

- Some of the included patients might not have been bleeding at the time
  of randomization. The authors recognized this limitation and showed an
  effect of tranexamic acid on mortality specifically from bleeding.
- While tranexamic acid reduced mortality it did not decrease the number
  of blood products used or the percentage of patients who needed
  transfusion, which raises questions with regard to the mechanism
  by which the drug worked. Hyperfibrinolysis is well documented in
  trauma patients, but one cannot be certain that the antibrinolytic effect
  of tranexamic acid resulted in its protective effect in the absence of
  difference in the rate of transfusion between the 2 groups.
- Conduct of the study in many moderate to low income countries led to
  controversy regarding the generalizability of its findings in high income
  countries with advanced trauma systems.
- Randomization was determined by "the uncertainty principle," i.e.,
  patients for whom the physician considered that there was a clear

indication for tranexamic acid were not randomly assigned nor were patients for whom there was considered to be a clear contraindication to tranexamic acid treatment. The use of the "uncertainty principle" for determining whether tranexamic acid was indicated administered without any use of laboratory studies confirming bleeding or coagulation status, has also been the subject of criticism.

Other Relevant Studies and Information: Shortly after the publication of the CRASH-2 Trial, The Military Application of Tranexamic Acid in Trauma Emergency Resuscitation (MATTERs) Study sought to retrospectively study the effect of tranexamic acid administration in the military setting. [2] Out of 896 consecutively admitted patients to a military hospital in Afghanistan, 293 had received tranexamic acid. The mortality of the tranexamic acid patients was significantly lower than that of the non-tranexamic acid patients (17.4% vs. 23.9%, respectively; p value = 0.03), despite having higher injury severity scores. This benefit was even more pronounced in the subgroup of patients who received massive transfusion (14.4% vs. 28.1%, respectively; p value = 0.004), where multivariable analysis confirmed that tranexamic acid was independently associated with more than 7-fold increase in survival. [2-4] Using the World Health Organization (WHO) mortality estimates and the results of the CRASH-2 trial, a separate 2012 study estimated that hundreds of thousands of trauma deaths could be avoided worldwide with a systematic use of tranexamic acid when hemorrhage is suspected. [5]

Recent consensus guidelines recommend the administration of tranexamic acid for the bleeding trauma patient:

- The European guideline on management of major bleeding and coagulopathy following trauma recommend that tranexamic acid be administered within 3 h after injury and suggest that protocols for the management of bleeding patients consider administration of the first dose of tranexamic acid en route to the hospital. [6]
- The ACS TQIP Best Practice Guidelines for Massive Transfusion recommend tranexemic acid administration in all injured patients that are actively bleeding and are within 3 h of injury. [7]

Summary and Implications: The early administration of the antifibrinolytic agent tranexamic acid, as a 1 gram load followed by a 1 gram infusion over 8 h, can reduce mortality among trauma patients who are experiencing bleeding without any apparent increase in vascular occlusion events.

CLINICAL CASE: USING TRANEXAMIC ACID IN A HYPOTENSIVE TRAUMA PATIENT PRESENTING FOLLOWING A HIGH SPEED MOTOR VEHICLE CRASH

Case History:

You are the intensivist on call in a busy level 1 trauma center. Your pager goes off: "STAT trauma, high speed motor vehicle crash, blood pressure 74/40, estimated time of arrival 5 min." The trauma surgeon suspects massive hemorrhage from a liver injury, and quickly transfers the patient to the operating room where an emergent damage control laparotomy is performed and the abdomen is packed. The patient reaches your intensive care unit 2 h following the initial injury and is still requiring blood product resuscitation. As the intensivist in charge, should you use tranexamic acid?

Suggested Answer:

The CRASH-2 trial provides robust level-one evidence for the use of tranexamic acid in trauma patients presenting with bleeding and signs of hemorrhagic shock. In that study, the absolute mortality decreased from 16.0% to 14.5% without any increase in vascular occlusive events. Furthermore, the benefit was most pronounced if tranexamic acid was administered within less than 3 h from the injury and in patients with systolic blood pressure less than 75 mm Hg.

This patient would be a perfect candidate for an immediate start of tranexamic acid in the intensive care unit, with 1 gram bolus followed by an infusion of 1 g over 8 h. Although tranexamic acid will not replace the presence of an experienced trauma team and a mature system that quickly recognize the hemorrhage, the need for surgical control of the hemorrhage, and the value of a damage control resuscitation/surgery strategy, there is little reason not to administer tranexamic acid and reap an additional 9–15% improved survival of this patient in extremis.

References

1. CRASH-2 trial collaborators; Shakur H, Roberts I, Bautista R, et al. Effects of tranexamic acid on death, vascular occlusive events, and blood transfusion in trauma patients with significant haemorrhage (CRASH-2): a randomised, placebo-controlled trial. *Lancet.* 2010; 376(9734):23–32.
2. Morrison JJ, Dubose JJ, Rasmussen TE, Midwinter MJ. Military Application of Tranexamic Acid in Trauma Emergency Resuscitation (MATTERs) study. *Arch Surg.* 2012;147(2):113–119.

3. Kaafarani HM, Velmahos GC. Damage control resuscitation in trauma. *Scand J Surg.* 2014;103(2):81–88.
4. Roberts I. Tranexamic acid in trauma: how should we use it? *J Thromb Haemost.* 2015;13(Suppl 1):S195–199.
5. Ker K, Kiriya J, Perel P, et al. Avoidable mortality from giving tranexamic acid to bleeding trauma patients. an estimation based on WHO mortality data, a systematic literature review and data from the CRASH-2 trial. *BMC Emerg Med.* 2012;12:3.
6. Rossaint R, Bouillon B, Cerny V, et al. The European guideline on management of major bleeding and coagulopathy following trauma: fourth edition. *Crit Care.* 2016;20:100.
7. https://www.facs.org/~/media/files/quality%20programs/trauma/tqip/massive%20transfusion%20in%20trauma%20guildelines.ashx. Last accessed 3/10/2017.

41

Transfusion of Plasma, Platelets, and Red Blood Cells in a 1:1:1 versus a 1:1:2 Ration and Mortality in Patients with Severe Trauma

The PROPPR Randomized Clinical Trial

YUK MING LIU AND KATHRYN BUTLER

"… early administration of plasma, platelets, and red blood cells in a 1:1:1 ratio compared with a 1:1:2 ration did not result in significant differences in mortality at 24 hours or at 30 days."

—THE PROPPR STUDY GROUP

Research Question: How effective and safe is rapid transfusion of patients with severe traumatic hemorrhage using plasma, platelets, and red blood cells in a 1:1:1 ratio compared to a 1:1:2 ratio?[1]

Funding: A grant US National Heart, Lung, and Blood Institute, and funding from the US Department of Defense, the Defence Research and Development Canada in partnership with the Canadian Institutes of Health Research

Year Study Began: August 2012

Year Study Published: December 2013

Study Location: 12 North American level 1 trauma centers

Who Was Studied: Patients 15 years or older, severely injured patients who met local criteria for highest level trauma activation. Patients were received directly from the scene of injury and received at least 1U of blood product in the pre-hospital setting or within 1 hour of arrival to hospital. These patients were also predicted to meet criteria for massive transfusion by the Assessment of Blood Consumption score[2] or physician judgment.

Who Was Excluded: Patients with the following characteristics: received > 3 units of red blood cells given before randomization, received > 5 consecutive minutes of CPR (with chest compressions) prior to arriving at the hospital or within the emergency department, received a lifesaving intervention from an outside hospital or health care facility, required a thoracotomy prior to receiving randomized blood products, directly admitted from a correctional facility, burns > 20% body surface area, suspected inhalation injury, pregnant, devastating injuries expected to die within 1 hour of admission, had a known DNR order prior to randomization, enrolled in a concurrent randomized clinical trial study.

How Many Patients: Initially 580 patients were planned, however the size was increased to 680 patients according to the trial's adaptive design.

Study Overview: See Figure 41.1 for an overview of the study design.

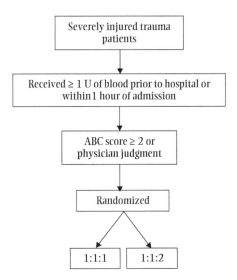

Figure 41.1 Summary of PROPPR Trial Design.

Study Intervention: Patients were randomized within each of the 12 study sites. The blood products were prepared by each site's blood bank and delivered to the bedside within 10 minutes. The initial container was sealed to blind the physicians to the treatment assignment. The 1:1:1 intervention group had 1 pack (average 6 units) of platelets, 6units of fresh frozen plasma (FFP) and 6 units of red blood cells (RBC). The products were transfused in the following order: platelets first followed by alternating RBC and FFP. For the 1:1:2 ratio control group, the initial and all odd numbered containers of products contained 3 units of FFP and 6 units of RBC and were transfused alternating 2 units RBC and 1 unit of FFP. The second and even number container of products contained 3units of FFP, 1 pack platelets, and 6 units of RBC. The platelets were given first followed by 2 units RBC and 1 unit of FFP.

Several criteria determined the discontinuation of transfusion products: achievement of hemostasis, death, declaration of treatment futility, no need for further blood products after randomization, and protocol violations.

Follow-up: 30 days.

Endpoints: Primary endpoints were 24-hour and 30-day all-cause mortality. Secondary outcomes included time to hemostasis, blood product volumes transfused, complications, hospital/ventilator/ICU-free days, incidence of surgical procedures, and functional status at hospital discharge or first 30days.

RESULTS

- There was no significant difference in mortality at 24 hours or at 30 days
  - 24 hours: 12.7% in the 1:1:1 group versus 17.0% in the 1:1:2 group ($p = 0.12$)
  - 30 days: 22.4% in the 1:1:1 group versus 26.1% in the 1:1:2 group ($p = 0.26$)
- The Kaplan-Meier survival curve showed a trend towards favoring 1:1:1 group which was not statistically significant
- A significantly higher number of patients achieved anatomic hemostasis in the 1:1:1 group compared with the 1:1:2 group with a P value = 0.006. However, the median time to achieve hemostasis did not differ between groups.
- More patients in the 1:1:1 group achieved hemostasis and fewer experienced death due to exsanguination by 24 hours.
- There were no notable differences in the rates of complications for the two groups, including acute respiratory distress syndrome, multi-organ failure, sepsis, and transfusion related complications.
- No differences were observed in any of the ancillary outcomes that were prespecified to evaluate for effectiveness and safety of the transfusion ratios (Table 41.1).

Table 41.1. Summary of PROPPR Trial Key Findings

Outcome	1:1:1	1:1:2	P value
24-hr mortality	12.7%	17%	0.12
30-day mortality	22.4%	26.1%	0.26
Exsanguination in first 24 hrs decreased	9.2%	14.6%	0.03
Time achieve hemostasis, median (min)	105	100	0.44

Criticisms and Limitations:

- Clinicians were unblinded after randomization by delivery of blood products from blood bank. Unblinding after the protocol started could potentially have resulted in bias in outcomes assessment.
- This study was appropriately powered to detect a 10% difference in mortality between the 1:1:1 and 1:1:2 groups; however, the study could not definitively establish a benefit < 10%. It is possible that a larger trial would have identified significant differences in outcomes between the groups.
- The timing of blood product administration was affected by the study protocol, with the 1:1:1 group likely receiving platelets earlier and the 1:1:2 group receiving plasma earlier.
- Only approximately 20% of patients with each group based received tranexamic acid an antifibrinolytic, which has been shown to be beneficial to limiting hemorrhage in severe trauma.[3,4] The effects of tranexamic acid use in combination with the transfusion ratios compared in this study is unclear.
- The study used the definition of "massive transfusion" as those patients requiring 10 or more units of RBCs in the first 24 hours. At least half the patients in their study did not reach this transfusion volume.

Other Relevant Studies and Information:

- Retrospective studies of massively transfused trauma patients demonstrated improved survival in patients transfused at a high FFP:RBC ratio as well as in those transfused at a high platelet:RBC ratio (i.e., ≥1:2).[5,6]
- The Prospective, Observational, Multicenter, Major Trauma Transfusion (PROMMTT) Study demonstrated that patients with ratios of plasma:RBC and platelets:RBC < 1:2 were more likely to die in the first 6 hours than patients with ratios ≥1:1.[7]
- Recent resuscitation guidelines from the Eastern Association for the Surgery of Trauma (EAST) and the American College of Surgeons Trauma Quality Improvement Program (ACS-TQIP) recommend high

plasma-to-RBC and platelet-to-RBC ratios as part of damage control resuscitation.[8,9]

Summary and Implications: A growing body of literature suggests that massive transfusion protocols confer mortality benefits for trauma patients in hemorrhagic shock; however, such protocols still require standardization. In the PROPPR trial, there was suggestion of improved hemostasis and less death from exsanguinations with a 1:1:1 transfusion ratio versus a 1:1:2 approach; however, the differences did not reach statistical significance, perhaps in part because the study was underpowered. Further trials are warranted.

CLINICAL CASE: RESUSCITATION GUIDED BY THE PROPPR TRIAL

Case History:

A 38-year-old male is transferred from the scene of a high-speed motorcycle collision with a tree. At the scene, the patient is unresponsive, and is intubated for airway protection. His vitals in the field are BP 92/60, HR 133, 95% saturation on 100% FiO_2. On presentation to the Emergency Department, his BP is now in the 80s/60s and HR remains in the 130s. He has received a liter of Lactated Ringer's. His injuries include severe flail chest, bilateral hemopneumothoraces with > 1.5 L blood on chest tube placement on the right. While a FAST is performed, one unit of blood is transfused with minimal change in the hemodynamics. The FAST study is positive for hemoperitoneum. Pelvis X-ray shows an open book fracture. The decision is made to proceed emergently to the operating room for thoracotomy, exploratory laparotomy, and external pelvic fixation with preperitoneal packing.

What principles should guide this patient's resuscitation perioperatively?

Suggested Answer:

Clinically, the patient has massive hemorrhage from trauma to the chest, abdomen and pelvis. Based on the PROPPR trial, the ABC scoring system is 3 and he would meet criteria for massive transfusion. Activation of the massive transfusion protocol would be reasonable for this patient and should continue in the OR. Based on the results of the PROPPR trial and subsequent recommendations, damage control resuscitation using high plasma-to-RBC and platelet-to-RBC should be employed. The need for continuation of the massive transfusion protocol should be determined by the hemodynamic response and evidence of ongoing bleeding.

References

1. Holcomb JB, et al. Transfusion of plasma, platelets, and red blood cells in a 1:1:1 vs a 1:1:2 ratio and mortality in patients with severe trauma: the PROPPR randomized clinical trial. *JAMA*. 2015;313(5):471–482.
2. Nunez TC, Voskresensky IV, Dossett LA, Shinall R, Dutton WD, Cotton BA. Early prediction of massive transfusion in trauma: simple as ABC (Assessment of Blood Consumption)? *J Trauma*. 2009;66(2):346–352.
3. CRASH-2 trial collaborators, et al., Effects of tranexamic acid on death, vascular occlusive events, and blood transfusion in trauma patients with significant haemorrhage (CRASH-2): a randomised, placebo-controlled trial. *Lancet*. 2010; 376(9734): 23–32.
4. Roberts I, Prieto-Merino D, Manno D. Mechanism of action of tranexamic acid in bleeding trauma patients: an exploratory analysis of data from the CRASH-2 trial. *Crit Care*. 2014;18(6):685.
5. Borgman MA, Spinella PC, Perkins JG, et al. The ratio of blood products transfused affects mortality in patients receiving massive transfusions at a combat support hospital. *J Trauma*. 2007;63:805.
6. Holcomb JB, Wade CE, Michalek JE, et al. Increased plasma and platelet to red blood cell ratios improves outcome in 466 massively transfused civilian trauma patients. *Ann Surg*. 2008;248:447.
7. Holcomb JB, et al. The PRospective Observational Multicenter Major Trauma Transfusion (PROMMTT) study. *J Trauma Acute Care Surg*. 2013;75(1 Suppl 1):S1–2.
8. Camazine MN, Hemmila MR, Leonard JC, et al. Massive transfusion policies at trauma centers participating in the American College of Surgeons Trauma Quality Improvement Program. *J Trauma Acute Care Surg*. 2015;78(6 Suppl 1):S48–53.
9. Cannon JW, Khan MA, Raja AS, et al. Damage control resuscitation in patients with severe traumatic hemorrhage: A practice management guideline from the Eastern Association for the Surgery of Trauma. *J Trauma Acute Care Surg*. 2017;82(3):605–617.

Infectious

42

Comparison of 8 versus 15 Days of Antibiotic Therapy for Ventilator-Associated Pneumonia in Adults

A Randomized Trial

LAURIE O. MARK AND JEAN KWO

"[F]or ICU patients who develop microbiologically proven VAP, we found no clinical advantage of prolonging antimicrobial therapy to 15 days compared with 8 days."

—CHASTRE ET AL.

Research Question: In adult patients with ventilator-associated pneumonia, is treatment with an 8-day course of antimicrobials as effective as a 15-day course?[1]

Funding: The Délégation à la Recherche Clinique, Assistance Publique-Hopitaux de Paris.

Year Study Began: 1999

Year Study Published: 2003

Study Location: 51 ICUs in France

Who Was Studied: Intubated ICU patients mechanically ventilated for at least 48 hours that were older than 18 years with a clinical suspicion for ventilator-associated pneumonia (VAP), had positive quantitative cultures of distal pulmonary secretion samples, and were started on empiric antimicrobial therapy within 24 hours of bronchoscopy.

Who Was Excluded: Patients who were pregnant, enrolled in another trial, had little chance of survival, neutropenic, had concomitant acquired immunodeficiency syndrome, received immunosuppressants or long-term corticosteroids, concomitant extrapulmonary infection that required antimicrobial therapy, or their attending physician declined to use full life support.

How Many Patients: 401

Study Overview: See Figure 42.1 for an overview of the study design.

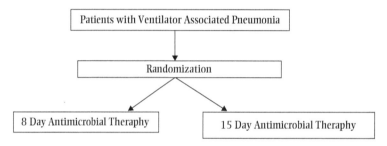

Figure 42.1 Summary of the study design.

Study Intervention: Patients were randomized to receive either 8 or 15 days of antibiotics. Antimicrobial therapy was left to the discretion of the treating physician. However, the preferred initial empiric antibiotic regimen consisted of an aminoglycoside or a fluoroquinolone, and a broad-spectrum beta-lactam antimicrobial agent. It was encouraged to narrow the initial regimen based on culture results. All antibiotics were discontinued at the end of day 8 or day 15, according to the randomization assignment unless there was a recurrence of pulmonary infection before that day or an infection preceding the VAP.

Follow-Up: 28 days after initial bronchoscopy

Endpoints: Primary outcomes: All-cause mortality after 28 days, microbiologic recurrence of pulmonary infection, and mean number of antibiotic-free days. Secondary outcomes: ventilator-free days, organ failure-free days, ICU days, progression of organ dysfunction scores from day 1 to day 28, rate of unfavorable outcomes (defined as death, infection recurrence, or prescription of new antibiotic treatment lasting longer than 48 hours for any reason), 60-day mortality, in-hospital mortality, and percentage of emerging multiresistant bacteria during the ICU stay.

RESULTS

- There was no difference in all-cause mortality between the 8-day and 15 day groups (18.8% vs. 17.2%) at 28 days after VAP onset.
- There was no difference in pulmonary infection recurrence between the 8-day and 15-day groups (28.9% vs. 26%) 28 days after VAP onset.
- Patients in the 8-day antimicrobial therapy group had significantly more antibiotic-free days than those in the 15-day group (13.1 vs. 8.7 days).
- There were no significant differences between the 8-day and 15-day groups in the numbers of patients who required a continuation of antimicrobials after the randomly assigned time course.
- In patients with primary pulmonary infections caused by nonfermenting gram-negative bacilli (i.e., *Pseudomonas aeruginosa, Acinetobacter baumannii and Stenotrophomonas maltophilia*), the 8-day group had a higher pulmonary infection recurrence rate than the 15-day group (40.6% vs. 25.4%).
- There were no significant differences between the 8-day and 15-day group in terms of secondary outcomes.
- Among the patients who developed recurrent pulmonary infections, those in the 8-day group were less likely to have multi-resistant pathogens than those in the 15-day group (Table 42.1).

Table 42.1. Summary of the Study's Key Findings

Outcome	8-Day Group	15-Day Group	Between Group Risk Difference (90% CI)
All-cause mortality	18.8%	17.2%	1.6 (−3.7 to 6.9)
Microbiologically documented pulmonary infection recurrence	28.9%	26%	2.9 (−3.2 to 9.1)
Antibiotic-free days	13.1	8.7	4.4 (3.1 to 5.6)

Criticisms and Limitations:

- It was uncertain whether that lack of blinding (after day 8) affected the results. However, double blinding after day 8 would have would have posed significant logistical problems such as finding an adequate placebo for the drugs and the inability to blind drugs when dosage adjustments were required to account for plasma concentration or renal function.
- The study excluded patients with early-onset pneumonia who had not previously received antibiotics, severely immunocompromised patients, patients with a low chance of survival, and patients whose initial

antimicrobial therapy was not appropriate. These exclusions limit the generalizability of these findings to other ICU populations.

Other Relevant Studies and Information:

- A prospective, randomized, controlled clinical trial by Micek et al.[2] involving 290 patients showed that implementation of an antibiotic discontinuation policy for clinically suspected VAP was safe and resulted in a decreased duration of antibiotic therapy.
- A systematic review and meta-analysis of short versus long-duration antibiotic regimens for VAP also found no difference in mortality with short duration antimicrobial therapy for VAP (7–8 days) compared with long-duration treatment (10–15 days).[3] While there was no statistical difference in relapses between the two groups, there was a trend toward lower relapses in the long-duration group.
- A 2015 Cochrane meta-analysis[4] concluded that a short course of antimicrobial therapy (7–8 days) might be more appropriate for patients with VAP than a prolonged course (10–15 days) because it did not increase the risk of adverse clinical outcomes and may reduce the emergence of resistant organisms. However, for patients with VAP due to nonfermenting gram-negative bacilli, short course therapy may be associated with a higher risk of recurrence. The quality of evidence was limited by the small number of studies, differences in patient populations, and differences in interventions and reported outcomes.
- A newer method to determine duration of antibiotic therapy is monitoring of serum biomarker levels such as procalcitonin, a good predictor of relapse.[5] Protocols implementing short course therapy durations with vigilance toward clinical response and procalcitonin levels may help reduce duration of antimicrobial therapy without negatively impacting outcomes.[6]
- Based on these and other findings, the American Thoracic Society recommends shortening duration of therapy for VAP from the traditional long-duration (8–15 days) to short duration (7 days).[7]

Summary and Implications: In ICU patients who develop microbiologically proven VAP, an 8-day antimicrobial course is not inferior to a 15-day course with respect to all-cause mortality or recurrence of pulmonary infection. These findings may not apply to patients who are immunocompromised as they were excluded from this study, or those with infections due to a nonfermenting gram-negative bacillus. In addition there may be situations in which a shorter or longer duration of antibiotics may be indicated, depending upon the rate of improvement of clinical, radiologic, and laboratory parameters.

CLINICAL CASE: 8 VERSUS 15 DAY COURSE OF ANTIMICROBIAL THERAPY FOR VENTILATOR ASSOCIATED PNEUMONIA

Case History:

A 60-year-old man who underwent an abdominal aortic aneurysm repair has been intubated on mechanical ventilation in the intensive care unit, for the past 5 days. He is febrile to 102°F, chest x-ray shows development of a new infiltrate in the left lower lobe, and purulent secretions are obtained from the endotracheal tube. Bronchoscopy is performed and cultures obtained. How should this patient be treated?

Suggested Answer:

Chastre et al.[1] showed that an 8-day course of antimicrobial therapy is not inferior to a 15-day course for the treatment of ventilator associated pneumonia. A lower respiratory culture has been obtained and now the patient should be started on empiric broad spectrum antibiotics. The American Thoracic Society's (ATS) guidelines for empiric antimicrobial therapy for HAP/VAP/HCAP in patients with late-onset disease (hospitalized for 5 days or more) or risk factors for multidrug-resistant pathogens include an antipseudomonal cephalosporin, or antipseudomonal carbepenem, or a beta-lactamase inhibitor plus an antipseudomonal fluoroquinolone, or aminoglycoside.[7] Vancomycin or Linezolid should also be started for empiric coverage of methicillin-resistant *Staphylococcus aureus*. The antibiotics should be modified or narrowed once the results of the respiratory tract cultures return. The antibiotic course should be set for 8 days unless the cultures are positive for a nonfermenting gram-negative bacillus, or the patient's initial antibiotic regimen was not appropriate for the causative microorganism. Clinical improvement (decreased white blood count, improved oxygenation, decreased fevers) should occur within 48 to 72 hours.[7] Failure to improve clinically by day 3 should prompt an evaluation for other organisms or drug-resistant organisms responsible for infection. The patient should also be evaluated for other nonpulmonary sources of infection and for complications for pneumonia and its therapy (e.g., pulmonary abscess, empyema).

References

1. Chastre J et al. Comparison of 8 vs 15 days of antibiotic therapy for ventilator-associated pneumonia in adults. *JAMA*. 2003;290:2588–2598.
2. Micek ST, et al. A randomized controlled trial of an antibiotic discontinuation policy for clinically suspected ventilator-associated pneumonia. *Chest*. 2004;125:1791–1799.

3. Dimopoulos G et al. Short- vs long-duration antibiotic regimens for ventilator-associated pneumonia: a systematic review and meta-analysis. *Chest.* 2013;144:1759–1767.

4. Pugh R et al. Short course versus prolonged-course antibiotic therapy for hospital-acquired pneumonia in critically ill adults. *Cochrane Database Syst Rev.* 2015;(8):CD007577.

5. Stolz D et al. Procalcitonin for reduced antibiotic exposure in ventilator-associated pneumonia: a randomized study. *Eur Resp J.* 2009;34: 1364–1375.

6. Schuetz P, Müller B, Christ-Crain M, et al. Procalcitonin to initiate or discontinue antibiotics in acute respiratory tract infections. *Cochrane Database Syst Rev.* 2012;(9):CD007498.

7. Kalil AC, Metersky ML, Klompas M, et al. Management of adults with hospital-acquired and ventilator-associated pneumonia: 2016 clinical practice guidelines by the Infectious Diseases Society of America and the American Thoracic Society. *Clin Infect Dis.* 2016;63:e61–e111.

43

Bronchoscopy with Bronchoalveolar Lavage versus Endotracheal Aspiration for the Diagnosis of Ventilator-Associated Pneumonia

SAMAD RASUL AND DAVID C. KAUFMAN

"Two diagnostic strategies for ventilator-associated pneumonia—bronchoalveolar lavage with quantitative culture of the bronchoalveolar-lavage fluid and endotracheal aspiration with nonquantitative culture of the aspirate—are associated with similar clinical outcomes and similar overall use of antibiotics."
— THE CANADIAN CRITICAL CARE TRIALS GROUP

Research Question: Does the diagnosis of ventilator-associated pneumonia by quantitative culture of bronchoalveolar lavage fluid or by non-quantitative culture of the endotracheal aspirate affect 28-day mortality rates?[1]

Funding: Grants from the Canadian Institutes of Health Research and Physicians' Services Incorporated of Ontario. Unrestricted grants from AstraZeneca and Bayer.

Year Study Began: May 2000

Year Study Published: 2006

Study Location: 28 ICUs in Canada and the United States

Who Was Studied: Immunocompetent adults receiving mechanical ventilation who had suspected ventilator-associated pneumonia after 4 days in the intensive care unit.

Who Was Excluded: Immunocompromised individuals: patients considered to be unsuitable for bronchoscopy; those allergic to study antibiotics; patients infected or colonized with Pseudomonas species or methicillin-resistant *Staphylococcus aureus*; recent recipients of study drugs (ciprofloxacin within 24 hours and meropenem within 7 days before enrollment); patients expected to die or undergo withdrawal of treatment within 72 hours after enrollment; those unlikely to leave the ICU within 3 weeks; pregnant or lactating women; or patients previously enrolled in this or another interventional trial.

Study Overview: Ventilator-associated pneumonia (VAP) is common, costly, and associated with increased morbidity and mortality. Diagnosis of VAP is based on clinical suspicion and microbiologic confirmation of a sample obtained from the lower respiratory tract. Debate exists regarding the best approach to sample lower respiratory tract secretions. The study by the Canadian Critical Care Trials Group (CCCTG) was designed to compare "invasive" (i.e., bronchoscopic BAL and quantitative cultures) and "noninvasive" (i.e., ETA and nonquantitative cultures) sampling techniques to diagnose VAP (Figure 43.1).

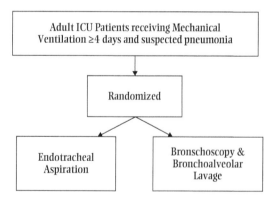

Figure 43.1 Summary of the study design.

How Many Patients: 740

Study Intervention: Patients receiving mechanical ventilation and suspected of having ventilator associated pneumonia after 4 days in the ICU were randomized to receive either bronchoscopy with quantitative culture of the bronchoalveolar lavage fluid or non-quantitative culture of endotracheal aspirate. Once diagnostic sampling was performed, subjects were randomly assigned to one of two empiric antibiotic regimens, meropenem and ciprofloxacin vs. meropenem alone, in a two-by-two factorial design. Antibiotics were then adjusted by the clinical team once culture results were known. If the culture showed no growth, study antibiotics were discontinued except in patients with a high pretest likelihood of ventilator-associated pneumonia.

Follow-up: 28 days or to hospital discharge

Endpoints: The primary outcome variable was the 28-day mortality rate. Secondary outcomes variables included survival in the ICU, discharge from the hospital, duration of mechanical ventilation, length of ICU and hospital stay, response to clinical and microbiologic treatment, organ-dysfunction score, and the use or nonuse of antibiotics after culture results were known.

RESULTS

- There was no significant difference in 28-day mortality between the bronchoalveolar-lavage group and the endotracheal aspiration group (18.9% vs. 18.4%; $P = 0.94$).
- There was no significant difference between the bronchoalveolar-lavage group and the endotracheal aspiration group in the time from randomization to discontinuation of mechanical ventilation (median 8.9 days vs. 8.8 days; $P = 0.31$), to discharge from the ICU (12.3 days vs. 12.2 days; $P = 0.22$) or to discharge from the hospital (40.2 vs. 47.0 days; $P = 0.13$).
- 59.7% patients in the bronchoalveolar lavage group had a positive culture compared to 51.9% in the endotracheal aspiration group ($P = 0.03$).
- Time from suspicion of ventilator associated pneumonia to initiation of study antibiotics was longer in the bronchoalveolar lavage group than in the endotracheal aspiration group (median 8.0 hours vs. 6.8 hours; $P < 0.001$).

Criticisms and Limitations:

- The investigators were aware of the study interventions and clinical judgement was involved in determining the pretest likelihood and final classification of ventilator associated pneumonia, which may have led to differential treatment.
- The prevalence of Pseudomonas species and methicillin resistant *Staphylococcus aureus* was only 6.4% and 1.6%, respectively; this rate is much lower than what has been observed by others.[2] Therefore,

the findings of this study may not be applicable in settings where
Pseudomonas and methicillin resistant *Staphylococcus aureus* are more
prevalent.

• The exclusion of patients known to be colonized with methicillin
resistant *Staphylococcus aureus* or pseudomonas species severely limits
the usefulness of the study's findings, since these are the pathogens
most commonly reported to cause ventilator-associated pneumonia.
Furthermore it is in this more difficult-to-treat population that the
invasive–quantitative techniques may be most useful.

Other Relevant Studies and Information:

• Randomized trials comparing invasive versus non-invasive approaches
have produced conflicting results. Three small ($n < 100$) single center
Spanish trials did not show any advantage of bronchoalveolar lavage
with quantitative cultures with respect to mortality or other clinical
outcomes when compared with culture obtained by endotracheal
aspiration.[3,4,5]

• A multi-center French study of 413 patients with suspected VAP
showed that an invasive sampling approach reduced 14-day mortality,
organ dysfunction, and antibiotic use.[6] However, the French trial
differed from the CCCTG trial in several important respects. In the
CCCTG trial, BAL fluid culture was considered positive if a potential
pathogen was isolated, regardless of the colony count, which probably
explains both the unexpected finding of a higher rate of positive BAL
fluid cultures and the very high proportion of patients (85%) classified
as having pneumonia. Furthermore, Gram stains were used in part to
initiate therapy and early cultures were used to adapt therapy in the
French trial, whereas all patients in the CCCTG trial received broad-
spectrum therapy for a median of 3 days.

• Recent clinical practice guidelines suggest endotracheal aspiration
with semiquantitative cultures to diagnose VAP, rather than invasive
sampling [i.e., bronchoalveolar lavage, protected specimen brush and
blind bronchial sampling (i.e., mini-BAL)] with quantitative cultures.[7]

Summary and Implications: Endotracheal aspiration with non-quantitative
culture of the aspirate to diagnose ventilator associated pneumonia leads to similar clinical outcomes and antibiotic use compared to those associated with bronchoalveolar lavage and quantitative culture of the bronchoalveolar lavage fluid. In
addition, bronchoscopy requires special training, is not universally available and
might delay treatment of ventilator associated pneumonia. Thus based on this
study, endotracheal aspiration with semiquantitative cultures is the suggested

method to diagnose VAP. Still, these findings may not apply to patients that are immunocompromised, those who are colonized with Pseudomonas species or methicillin resistant *Staphylococcus aureus*, or those who are pregnant or lactating, all of whom were excluded from this study.

CLINICAL CASE: DIAGNOSIS OF VENTILATOR ASSOCIATED PNEUMONIA

Case History:

A 70-year-old woman was admitted 5 days ago to the ICU after a fall with a subsequently diagnosed subdural hematoma and seizure. She was intubated on admission due to encephalopathy. On day 5 she was found to be febrile to 39°C with worsening hypoxemia and moderate amounts purulent appearing as green secretions in her endotracheal tube. Her white blood cell count was 14.5 x 10³ per µL and her chest x-ray reveals a new right basilar, dense consolidation. She is not in shock and her vital signs are stable. She is not colonized with Pseudomonas species or methicillin resistant *Staphylococcus aureus* and in this particular ICU, the prevalence of infection with these organisms and other multidrug resistant organisms is less than 10%. Based on the results of this trial, what diagnostic modality should be used to diagnose ventilator associated pneumonia?

Suggested Answer:

This patient has a high clinical pre-test likelihood of having ventilator associated pneumonia and should undergo diagnostic studies to pursue targeted antimicrobial therapy. She is not immunocompromised and is not colonized with Pseudomonas species or methicillin resistant *Staphylococcus aureus*. Since she is hemodynamically stable, there is an opportunity to obtain adequate specimen for a microbiological diagnosis. The results of the Canadian Critical Care Group Trial study suggest that there would be no additional benefit offered by a bronchoscopy with quantitative culture of the bronchoalveolar lavage fluid in terms of either 28 day mortality, or targeted antimicrobial therapy. Furthermore, there may be no advantage in terms of shortening the duration of mechanical ventilation or length of ICU or total hospital stay by pursuing bronchoscopy with quantitative culture of the bronchoalveolar lavage fluid. Therefore it is reasonable to send an endotracheal aspirate for non-quantitative culture. She should then be started on empirical antibiotics to treat ventilator associated pneumonia according to local epidemiological data and protocols. Her antimicrobial regimen should be adjusted according to the results of the culture and her clinical course.

References

1. The Canadian Critical Care Trials Group. A Randomized Trial of Diagnostic Techniques for Ventilator Associated Pneumonia. *N Eng J Med.* 2006; 355(25):2619–2630.
2. Kollef MH, Morrow LE, Niederman MS, et al. Clinical characteristics and treatment patterns among patients with ventilator-associated pneumonia. *Chest.* 2006;129(5):1210–1218.
3. Sanchez-Nieto JM, Torres A, Garcia- Cordoba F, et al. Impact of invasive and noninvasive quantitative culture sampling on outcome of ventilator-associated pneumonia: a pilot study. *Am J Respir Crit Care Med.* 1998;157:371–376. [Erratum, *Am J Respir Crit Care Med.* 1998;157:1005.]
4. Ruiz M, Torres A, Ewig S, et al. Noninvasive versus invasive microbiological investigation in ventilator associated pneumonia: evaluation of outcome. *Am J Respir Crit Care Med.* 2000;162:119–125.
5. Sole Violan J, Fernandez JA, Benitez AB, et al. Impact of quantitative invasive diagnostic techniques in the management and outcome of mechanically ventilated patients with suspected pneumonia. *Crit Care Med.* 2000;28:2737–2741.
6. Fagon JY, Chastre J, Wolff M, et al. Invasive and noninvasive strategies for management of suspected ventilator-associated pneumonia: a randomized trial. *Ann Intern Med.* 2000;132:621–630.
7. Kalil AC, Metersky ML, Klompas M, et al. Management of adults with hospital-acquired and ventilator associated pneumonia: 2016 clinical practice guidelines by the Infectious Diseases Society of America and the American Thoracic Society. *Clin Infect Dis.* 2016;63:e61–e111.

44

Randomized Trial of Combination versus Monotherapy for the Empiric Treatment of Suspected Ventilator-Associated Pneumonia

KIMBERLY POLLOCK AND ANGELA MEIER

"In immunocompetent critically ill patients, we observed that when broad-spectrum antibiotics are used for initial empirical therapy for clinically suspected late Ventilator Associated Pneumonia (VAP) in the setting of a low prevalence of high risk organisms outcomes appear similar whether combination therapy or monotherapy is used."

—HEYLAND ET AL.

Research Question: Does maximizing initial therapy using 2 antibiotics improve clinical outcomes compared with monotherapy in the treatment of suspected VAP?[1]

Sponsor: Grants from the Canadian Institutes of Health Research and Physicians Services Inc. of Ontario and unrestricted grants from AztraZeneca Inc. and Bayer Inc., Ontario Canada.

Year Study Began: 2000

Year Study Published: 2008

Study Location: 28 intensive care units in Canada and the United States

Who Was Studied: 740 adult patients who were mechanically ventilated for 96 hours and developed suspected pneumonia while intubated. Suspected pneumonia was defined by the presence of new or persistent radiographic features suggestive of pneumonia and two or more of the following: fever 38°C, leukocytosis (> 11.0×10^9 /L) or neutropenia (< 3.5×10^9 /L), purulent endotracheal aspirate secretions, isolation of pathogenic bacteria from the endotracheal aspirates, and increasing oxygen requirements.

Who Was Excluded: Patients who were immunocompromised; already colonized in the respiratory tract or infected with an organism not sensitive to study drugs (pseudomonas, MRSA), patients with an anticipated ICU stay of > 3 weeks or < 24 hours, patients deemed to be unsuitable candidates for bronchoscopy, patients with anaphylaxis to penicillin, cephalosporins or carbapenems, and patients who were pregnant or lactating. Patients who had received carbapenems or ciprofloxacin within 7 days of enrollment and patients who had received any antibiotic for the current suspicion of VAP.

How Many Patients: 371 were randomized to the monotherapy group and 396 were randomized to the combination therapy group.

Study Overview: See Figure 44.1 for an overview of the study design.

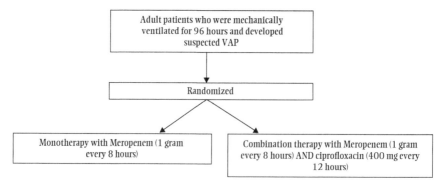

Figure 44.1 Summary of the study design.

Study Intervention: Patients were allocated to receive either Meropenem (1 gram every 8 hours) *and* ciprofloxacin (400 mg every 12 hours) *or* Meropenem alone (1 gram every 8 hours). Review of culture results was standardized and physicians were instructed to target their therapy and adjust antibiotic treatment based on culture data, specifically to administer a "single antibiotic with the narrowest spectrum that had activity against the infecting organism."[1] If pseudomonas species were isolated, 2 antibiotics with anti pseudomonal activity were recommended. Antibiotics were discontinued if culture results were negative except in patients with the highest pretest probability.

Follow-Up: 28 days (primary outcome)

Endpoints: Primary outcome was 28 day all-cause mortality. Secondary outcomes included: duration of mechanical ventilation, ICU length of stay, hospital length of stay, clinical and microbiological treatment response, antibiotic use, emergence of resistant organisms, rates of infection due to Clostridium difficile, and fungal colonization.

RESULTS

- Overall mortality at 28 days was 18.7%. There was no difference in 28-day mortality between the combination and monotherapy groups (relative risk = 1.05, 95% confidence interval 0.78–1.42, p = .74) (Table 44.1).

Table 44.1. KEY FINDINGS

Outcome	Result	P Value
Mortality at 28 Days	No difference between groups	0.74
Resistance:	9.1% Combo group	0.99
	9.3% Mono group	
Clostridium difficile isolated from stool	5.4% Combo group	0.65
	7.6% Mono group	
Median time to discontinuation of mechanical ventilation alive	8.7 days Combo group	0.79
	9.3 days Mono group	
Discharge from ICU alive	12.1 days Combo group	0.84
	12.8 days Mono group	
Discharge from hospital alive	45.8 days Combo group	0.49
	39.1 Mono group	
Rates of colonization of sputum	Not statistically significant between the 2 groups	N/a
Proportion of patients who received adequate initial antibiotics	93.1% Combo group	0.01
	85.1% Mono group	

- Duration of intensive care unit and hospital stay, clinical and microbiological treatment response, emergence of antibiotic-resistant bacteria, isolation of Clostridium difficile in stool, and fungal colonization were also similar in the two groups.
- The proportion of patients who received adequate initial antibiotics was significantly greater in the combination group than in the monotherapy

group (93.1% vs. 85.1%, p = .01). Reasons for inadequate initial therapy were related to the presence of multidrug-resistant gram-negative bacteria such as Pseudomonas species, Acinetobacter species, Stenotrophomonas maltophilia, and MRSA in the enrollment cultures.

- In a subgroup of patients who had infection due to Pseudomonas species, Acinetobacter species, and multidrug-resistant gram-negative bacilli at enrollment, the adequacy of initial antibiotics (84.2% vs. 18.8%, p < .001) and microbiological eradication of infecting organisms (64.1% vs. 29.4%, p = .05) was higher in the combination group compared with the monotherapy group, but there were no differences in clinical outcomes.

- A prespecified subgroup analysis which compared the efficacy of combination therapy with monotherapy in patients with Pseudomonas species, Acinetobacter species, and multidrug-resistant Gram-negative bacteria revealed a trend toward greater eradication of the infecting organisms, shorter duration of ventilation and ICU stay, and lower ICU and hospital mortality with combination therapy. However, this subgroup analysis was underpowered to demonstrate statistical significance.

Criticisms and Limitations:

- The study was unblinded which may have resulted in differential treatment of the groups or the differential assessment of outcomes.
- Patients excluded in the study included those already colonized or infected in the respiratory tract with an organism not susceptible to one of the study drugs patients who were immunocompromised, had previously received one of the study antimicrobials, or had chronic disease. These excluded patients are more likely to be infected with antibiotic-resistant pathogens and may have provided better insight into the limitations of the antimicrobial regimens studied.
- The overall prevalence of Pseudomonas, MRSA, and other difficult to-treat organisms was low compared with other reports in the literature and may explain why the overall study results showed no difference in clinical outcomes. Therefore, this study does answer the question if VAP should be treated with mono or combination therapy in hospital settings with higher prevalence of multi-resistant organisms.
- The choice of antibiotics used in the study is questionable. According to American Thoracic Society/Infectious Diseases Society of America (ATS/IDSA) guidelines, these patients should have been treated with narrower spectrum monotherapy. Instead, patients were randomized to

a meropenem, which is much broader than recommended for patients without risk factors for MDR pathogen. Therefore the study does not validate whether narrow spectrum monotherapy can be used in patients without overt risk factors for MDR pathogens.

Other Relevant Studies and Information:

- The initial use of combination therapy for infections with Gram-negative bacteria is often justified by one of the following three reasons: (1) to ensure that the pathogen is adequately covered by at least one of the two components of the regimen), (2) to exploit the synergy between two antibiotic agents, or (3) to prevent or delay the emergence of resistance during antimicrobial therapy.[2]
- A large recent meta-analysis comparing monotherapy to multiple antibiotic therapies for VAP did not find a difference between monotherapy and combination therapy for the treatment of people with VAP.[3] However, since the contained studies did not identify patients with increased risk for multidrug-resistant bacteria, these data may not be generalizable to all patient groups. Due to lack of studies, we could not evaluate the best antibiotic choice for VAP, but carbapenems as a class may result in better clinical cure than other tested antibiotics.
- For patients at risk of multidrug resistant gram negative infections, including patients with compromised immune systems, those with previous ICU admissions, or recent recipients of broad-spectrum antibiotics, empiric antimicrobial treatment should include coverage of pathogens that may be resistant to previously administered antibiotics, and empiric combination therapy may be appropriate. However, in attempts to avoid further emergence of resistance and adverse side effects such as *C. difficile* infection, nephrotoxicity, and ototoxicity, the antimicrobial regimen should be promptly narrowed or discontinued based on the patient's clinical course and culture and susceptibility profile results.
- Clinical Practice Guidelines by the Infectious Diseases Society of America and the American Thoracic Society 2016 recommend that empiric coverage for VAP should include an at least 2 agents active against gram-negative organisms, including P. aeruginosa unless local or regional data suggest a low antibiotic resistance rates among gram-negatives, then a single agent is likely adequate.[4] This recommendation is based on national and international surveillance data suggest that

a considerable proportion of VAP is attributable to resistant gram-negatives organisms.

Summary and Implications: For critically ill patients who have suspected late VAP and are at low risk for difficult to treat gram-negative bacteria, the study and related evidence suggest that monotherapy is associated with similar outcomes compared with combination therapy. For those patients at high risk of difficult to treat gram-negative bacteria, some evidence suggests that combination therapy may be superior, although the impact and clinical outcomes are still uncertain.

CLINICAL CASE: TREATMENT OF VAP IN THE ICU

Case History:
Your hospital has a moderate sized ICU with 24 beds and very low prevalence of multi-resistant organisms such as MRSA and Pseudomonas. Based on the results of this study, should you recommend combination therapy for your patients if they are deemed to be low risk for difficult to treat gram-negative organisms?

Suggested Answer:
This study suggests that there is no difference in outcomes in patients with ventilator associated pneumonia treated with monotherapy vs. combination therapy if there is low risk for difficult-to-treat gram-negative bacteria. It suggests; however, that there may be a benefit in combination therapy when treating those suspected of having a multi-drug resistant organism on presentation. It is important to note that the mortality rate is increased with delays in effective antimicrobial treatment in critically ill patients and therefore initiation of broad-spectrum antibiotics may be prudent, which often means combination therapy. Furthermore in patients with compromised immune systems, those with previous ICU admissions or recent recipients of broad-spectrum antibiotics, empiric antimicrobial treatment should include coverage of pathogens that may be resistant to previously administered antibiotics, and empiric combination therapy may be appropriate.

In order to avoid further emergence of resistance and adverse side effects, the antimicrobial regimen should be promptly narrowed or discontinued based on the patient's clinical course and culture and susceptibility profile results. Overall, it is important to recognize infection early, empirically treat with an antibiotic that targets the most likely pathogen, and de-escalate antibiotics once cultures and sensitivities are identified.

References

1. Heyland DK, Dude P, Muscedere J, Day A, Cook D. Randomized trial of combination versus monotherapy for the empiric treatment of suspected ventilator-associated pneumonia. *Critical Care Med.* 2008;36(3):737–744.
2. Tama P, Cosgrove S, Maragakis L. Combination therapy for treatment of infections with gram-negative bacteria. *Clin Microbial Rev.* 2012;25(3):450–470.
3. Arthur LE, Kisoro RS, Salim AG, van Drivel ML, Sloane L. Antibiotics for ventilator-associated pneumonia. *Cochrane Database Sits Rev.* 2016;10:CD004267.
4. Kalil AC, Metersky ML, Klompas M, et al. Management of adults with hospital-acquired and ventilator-associated pneumonia: 2016clinical practice guidelines by the Infectious Diseases Society of America and the American Thoracic Society. *Clin Infect Dis.* 2016;63(5):e61–e111.

45

Use of Procalcitonin to Reduce Patients' Exposure to Antibiotics in Intensive Care Units (PRORATA Trial)

A Multicenter Randomized Controlled Trial

ALICE GALLO DE MORAES AND DANTE SCHIAVO

"A procalcitonin-guided strategy to treat suspected bacterial infections in non-surgical patients in intensive care units could reduce antibiotic exposure and selective pressure with no apparent adverse outcomes."
—BOUADMA ET AL.

Research Question: Does a procalcitonin (PCT)-based strategy to treat suspected bacterial infections in ICU patients reduce antibiotic exposure without adverse outcomes?[1]

Sponsors: Assistance Publique-Hôpitaux de Paris, France, and Brahms, Germany

Year Study Began: 2007

Year Study Published: 2010

Study Location: Five medical, two surgical ICUs in university-affiliated hospitals, and one medical-surgical ICU in a general hospital, totaling 140 ICU beds

Who Was Studied: Adults admitted with suspected infection were eligible for inclusion if they were not receiving antibiotics for more than 24 hours before inclusion. Patients who developed sepsis during their ICU stay were also eligible for enrollment.

Who Was Excluded: Patients younger than 18 years of age; pregnant women; patients with expected ICU stay of less than 3 days; patients with bone marrow transplant or chemotherapy-induced neutropenia; patients with infections requiring long-term antibiotic treatment (infective endocarditis, for example); those with a simplified acute physiologic score (SAPS II) of more than 65 points at inclusion; and patients with a do-not-resuscitate order.

How Many Patients: A total of 1315 patients were assessed for eligibility. Of those, 630 were enrolled and randomized, and a total of 621 were included in the analysis.

Study Overview: A prospective, randomized open-label multicenter trial was conducted. After baseline screening, patients were randomly assigned to either the PCT or the control group, in a 1:1 fashion, stratified by center (Figure 45.1). Investigators were masked to assignment before, but not after randomization. Patients were analyzed in an intention-to-treat protocol.

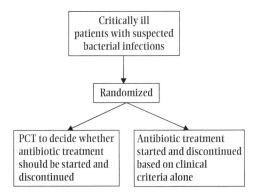

Figure 45.1 Summary of the PRORATA trial : implementation of an algorithm based on procalcitonin levels to guide antibiotics initiation, continuation and discontinuation in several ICU's was associated with less days of antibiotic use, without affecting mortality, LOS in the hospital or ICU and without generating the emergence of multi-resistant bacteria.

Study Intervention:

- *Procalcitonin Group:* Baseline PCT was used to decide if antibiotics should be started or not. When antibiotics were not initially started, physicians were advised to repeat clinical assessment and PCT measurements 6–12 hours later in order to detect a late PCT peak. If the clinical situation required immediate antibiotic administration (purulent meningitis or septic shock, for example), physicians were encouraged to start antibiotics prior to PCT results. PCT was assessed daily and used to decide if antibiotics should be continued or not (Figure 45.2).

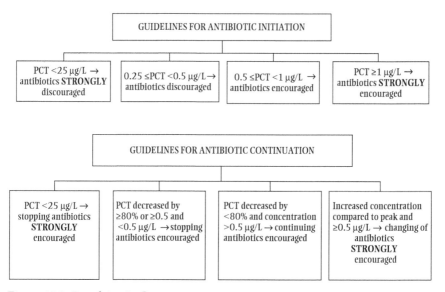

Figure 45.2 Procalcitonin Group.

- *Control group:* Initiation and duration of treatment was based on clinical judgment.
- *Both groups:* Drug selection was at the discretion of the treating physician.

Follow-Up: 12 months

Endpoints:

- *Primary:* mortality at days 28 and 60; number of days without antibiotics by day 28 after inclusion.
- *Secondary:* rates of relapse or superinfection; number of days without mechanical ventilation (MV); SOFA score; length of stay (LOS) in the ICU and hospital; days of antibiotic exposure; appearance of multidrug resistant bacteria.

RESULTS

The PCT group had more days without antibiotics at day 28 after inclusion, fewer days of antibiotics exposure per 1000 inpatient days and shorter duration of antibiotic treatment than the control group, without difference in mortality at day 28 or 60 (Table 45.1).

Table 45.1. SUMMARY OF SIGNIFICANT RESULTS

	Procalcitonin Group ($n = 307$)	Control Group ($n = 314$)	Between-Group Absolute Difference	P Value
28-Day mortality	65 (21.2%)	64 (20.4%)	0.8% (−4.6 to 6.2)	NA
60 Day mortality	92 (30.0%)	82 (26.1%)	3.8% (−2.1 to 9.7)	NA
Number of days without antibiotics	14.3 (9.1)	11.6 (8.2)	2.7 (1.4 to 4.1)	<0.0001
Days of antibiotic exposure per 1000 inpatient days	653	812	−159 (−185 to −131)	<0.0001
Duration of first episode of antibiotic treatment in the overall population (days [SD])	6.1 (6.0)	9.9 (7.1)	−3.8 (−4.8 to −2.7)	<0.0001

There was no difference between the groups in terms of relapse or superinfection, SOFA score, LOS in the ICU or hospital, and percentage of patients with emerging multi-drug-resistant organisms.

Criticisms and Limitations:

- The trial had an open-label design in which the treating physicians were aware of group assignment. Thus whether the procalcitonin concentrations themselves or simply the act of measuring procalcitonin led to the recorded reduction in antibiotic use is difficult to establish.
- Surgical patients represented only 10% of the study's total cohort, thus extrapolation of the results to the surgical population should be made with caution.
- In the procalcitonin group, the algorithm (Figure 45.2) was not followed in 53% of patients, either because the treating physician overruled it or because patients were discharged from the ICU and serial PCT measurements was not performed.
- While not statistically significant, a slightly higher number of patients in the procalcitonin group died between 29 and 60 days, potentially questioning the safety of the proposed protocol to limit the use of antibiotics in the ICU.
- In the procalcitonin group, antibiotics were encouraged for procalcitonin concentrations above 0·5 µg/L. However elevated concentrations of procalcitonin may be found in some patients without acute infections (e.g., patients receiving granulocyte transfusions, patients with acute graft-versus-host disease or liver metatstasis). Therefore, procalcitonin should not be considered as an accurate marker of infection in patients who fall into the above categories, and a procalcitonin-guided strategy could result in treatment excess.

Other Relevant Studies and Information:

- In a secondary analysis from a prospective study performed across 148 ICUs in Spain, median values of PCT were significantly higher in patients with A1N1 and concomitant community acquired bacterial and fungal coinfection (2).
- While PCT may be associated with bacterial infection in ICU patients, its diagnostic precision as a biomarker of infection remains problematic. Three meta-analysis performed on the subject have yielded conflicting results (3–5). The most recent analyzed 3244 patients from 30 studies, finding high heterogeneity between studies. The overall optimal threshold of 1.1 ng/mL to detect bacterial sepsis yield a mean sensitivity of 77% [95% confidence interval (CI) 72–81%] and mean specificity of 79% (95% CI 74–84%; 5).
- A smaller prospective, single center, single blind study corroborated the PRORATA trial results. Najafi et al showed a significant reduction in antibiotics use without significant changes in clinical outcomes, ICU and hospital LOS or mortality (6).
- Current consensus guidelines suggest using PCT levels plus clinical criteria to guide the discontinuation of antibiotic therapy, rather than clinical criteria alone (7).

Summary and Implications: This study suggests that managing critically ill patients with a PCT-guided antibiotic strategy to treat suspected bacterial infections results in more antibiotic-free days than those managed by clinical guidelines alone. Furthermore the mortality of patients in the PCT arm was non-inferior to those in the control group at day 28 and at day 60, using 10% as the margin of non-inferiority. This strategy could be beneficial for reducing antibiotic resistance in the ICU.

CLINICAL CASE: USE OF PROCALCITONIN TO GUIDE ANTIBIOTIC USE IN THE ICU

Case History:
You are admitting a patient from the community with sepsis but not in shock. Should you order procalcitonin prior to starting antibiotics?

Suggested Answer:
The PRORATA trial suggests that the measurement of PCT in ICU patients who were not in shock and did not have formal indications for immediate administration of antibiotics received fewer days of antibiotics. Despite days of antibiotic exposure being fewer in the procalcitonin group, mortality, ICU and hospital LOS were similar between the procalcitonin and control groups.

There is still controversy regarding the use of PCT as a diagnostic biomarker. The PRORATA study suggests that using an algorithm adding PCT measurement to history, exam, clinical, and diagnostic findings reduces the overall antibiotic exposure for adults in the ICU without adversely effecting mortality, LOS or drug resistance.

References

1. Bouadma L, Luyt CE, Tubach F, et al. Use of procalcitonin to reduce patients' exposure to antibiotics in intensive care units (PRORATA trial): a multicentre randomised controlled trial. *Lancet*. 2010;375(9713):463–474.
2. Rodriguez AH, Aviles-Jurado FX, Diaz E, et al. Procalcitonin (PCT) levels for ruling-out bacterial coinfection in ICU patients with influenza: A CHAID decision-tree analysis. *J Infect*. 2016;72(2):143–151.
3. Tang BM, Eslick GD, Craig JC, McLean AS. Accuracy of procalcitonin for sepsis diagnosis in critically ill patients: systematic review and meta-analysis. *Lancet. Infects Dis.* 2007;7(3):210–217.
4. Uzzan B, Cohen R, Nicolas P, Cucherat M, Perret GY. Procalcitonin as a diagnostic test for sepsis in critically ill adults and after surgery or trauma: a systematic review and meta-analysis. *Crit Care Med*. 2006;34(7):1996–2003.
5. Wacker C, Prkno A, Brunkhorst FM, Schlattmann P. Procalcitonin as a diagnostic marker for sepsis: a systematic review and meta-analysis. *Lancet. Infect Dis.* 2013;13(5):426–435.
6. Najafi A, Khodadadian A, Sanatkar M, et al. The comparison of procalcitonin guidance administer antibiotics with empiric antibiotic therapy in critically ill patients admitted in intensive care unit. *Acta Med Iranica*. 2015;53(9):562–567.
7. Kalil AC, Metersky ML, Klompas M, et al. Management of adults with hospital-acquired and ventilator associated pneumonia: 2016 clinical practice guidelines by the Infectious Diseases Society of America and the American Thoracic Society. *Clin Infect Dis*. 2016;63(5):e61–e111.

46

Nasopharyngeal and Oropharyngeal Decontamination to Prevent Nosocomial Infection in Cardiac Surgery Patients

JOSE L. DIAZ-GOMEZ AND SARAH W. ROBISON

"Decontamination of the nasopharynx and oropharynx with chlorhexidine gluconate appears to be an effective method to reduce nosocomial infection after cardiac surgery."

—SEGERS ET AL.

Research Question: Does routine decontamination of the nasopharynx and oropharynx with chlorhexidine gluconate reduce nosocomial infections after cardiac surgery?[1]

Sponsor: None. All materials were provided by the local hospital pharmacy.

Study Dates: August 1, 2003 through September 1, 2005

Year Study Published: 2006

Study Location: Single center 480-bed community hospital in Amsterdam, the Netherlands

Who Was Studied: Adult patients scheduled to undergo cardiac surgical procedures. The hospital performs 1200 of these procedures annually.

Who Was Excluded: Patients who underwent emergency procedures, those with preoperative infections or who were on antibiotics preoperatively (not prophylaxis), those with hypersensitivity to chlorhexidine gluconate, those treated with an alternative decontamination regimen, and patients hospitalized for less than 24 hours prior to surgery

How Many Patients: 991

Study Overview: Patients undergoing cardiac surgery with sternotomy were randomized, in a double-blind, placebo-controlled clinical trial to receive either chlorhexidine for nasopharyngeal and oropharyngeal decontamination or placebo (Figure 46.1).

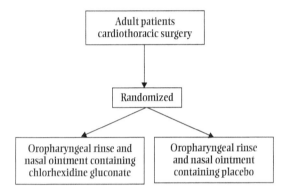

Figure 46.1 Summary of the study design.

Study Intervention: Patients assigned to the chlorhexidine group received a 0.12% chlorhexidine gluconate oral rinse and a 0.12% chlorhexidine gluconate gel for nasal application or to the placebo group where they received an oral rinse and topical gel of similar color, taste, and smell. Patients in the placebo group were dispensed placebos in identical packaging. In both groups, oropharyngeal solution (10 mL) was used as a mouth rinse and applied to buccal, pharyngeal, gingival, and tooth surfaces for 30 seconds 4 times daily. The nasal ointment was applied 4 times a day in both nostrils. The protocol was continued until the nasogastric tube was removed. All patients were treated according to the existing local open heart surgery protocol including showering with chlorhexidine gluconate soap, hair removal with electric clippers, and prophylactic antibiotics.

Follow-Up: 30 days

Endpoints:

- The *primary endpoint* was the overall incidence of nosocomial infection. Nosocomial infections were diagnosed following guidelines from the Centers for Disease Control and Prevention.

- *Secondary endpoints*:
  - Incidence of lower respiratory tract infections and incidence of surgical site infections
  - *S. aureus* nasal colonization
  - Use of therapeutic antimicrobials
  - Duration of hospital stay and in-hospital mortality
  - Adverse effect of trial medications

RESULTS

- There was a statistically significant reduction in the incidence of nosocomial infections in the group that underwent chlorhexidine decontamination compared to the placebo group. The intervention conferred an absolute risk reduction for nosocomial infections of 6.4%. Sixteen (number needed to treat) patients would have to receive oropharyngeal and nasopharyngeal decontamination with chlorhexidine gluconate to prevent one nosocomial infection.
- Only one reported adverse effect was reported with use of chlorhexidine gluconate. One patient reported temporary discoloration of the teeth.

Criticism and Limitations: This study examined a very specific patient population and was performed in one community hospital in the Netherlands. Findings may not be generalized to other institutions and countries.

Two methods of decontamination were simultaneously implemented in this study. It cannot be determined if one method (nasal chlorhexidine gel versus oral chlorhexidine solution) was more effective than the other, or if using one method alone would be sufficient to decrease the rates of nosocomial infection.

Other Relevant Studies and Information:

- Ten years prior to the study by Segers et al, a group in Indiana conducted a prospective, randomized, double-blind, placebo-controlled study using chlorhexidine solution for oral decontamination in patients undergoing cardiovascular surgery. They observed a statistically significant 69% reduction in the total number of respiratory infections in the treatment group.[2] Another group in Texas compared chlorhexidine gluconate solution and Listerine® (Johnson and Johnson, New Brunswick, NJ, USA) for oral decontamination in cardiac surgery patients. They found a reduced incidence of nosocomial pneumonia in chlorhexidine-treated patients; however, the results were not statistically significant. Their sample size was much smaller than the study by Segers et al and therefore may have been underpowered to detect a difference between groups.[3]

- A large, randomized, placebo-controlled, double-blind trial conducted at an academic center in the US compared the preoperative use of topical mupirocin to placebo for decontamination of the nares. Despite enrolling over 4000 patients in the study, they found no statistically significant difference in the overall incidence of nosocomial infection. However, the data did show that there was a significant decrease in the incidence of S. aureus nosocomial infections in patients with culture-positive colonization of S. aureus in the nares prior to decontamination.[4] One of the primary reasons chlorhexidine gel was used for nasopharyngeal decontamination in the Segers et al study (as opposed to mupirocin) was because there does not appear to be a risk for microbial resistance to chlorhexidine.[1,5]

- Regular oral care with chlorhexidine gluconate has become standard practice for the prevention of ventilator associated pneumonia (VAP) in most hospitals and the inclusion of regular oral care with chlorhexidine is part of the ventilator care bundle of the Institute for Healthcare Improvement.[6] However a recent meta-analysis concluded that while oral care with chlorhexidine prevents nosocomial pneumonia in cardiac surgery patients it may not decrease the incidence of ventilator-associated pneumonia risk in non-cardiac surgery patients.[7] In contrast a more recent metaanalysis of 18 randomized controlled trials of critically ill patients receiving mechanical ventilation for at least 48 hours concluded that chlorhexidine mouth rinse or gel, as part of oral hygiene care, reduces the risk of VAP compared to placebo or usual care from 25% to about 19% (P = 0.002).[8] There were no differences mortality, duration of mechanical ventilation or ICU length or stay in either study.

Summary and Implication: The results of this study and others suggest that use of chlorhexidine gluconate for oropharyngeal and nasopharyngeal decontamination is beneficial for reducing nosocomial infection in patients undergoing elective, nonemergent cardiovascular surgery. However chlorhexidine may not decrease the incidence of ventilator-associated pneumonia risk in non-cardiac surgery patients.

CLINICAL CASE: DECONTAMINATION IN ELECTIVE CARDIAC SURGERY

Case History:
A 66-year-old man is admitted on the day of surgery for elective minimally invasive cardiac surgery. Should he receive nasal and oropharyngeal decontamination with topical chlorhexidine?

Suggested Answer:

The results of this study and others suggest that topical chlorhexidine is beneficial for reducing nosocomial infection in patients undergoing elective, cardiovascular surgery. While the clinical characteristics of this patient's surgery differ somewhat (e.g., same day admission, minimally invasive surgery) from the patients enrolled in the study the low cost of treatment and minimal side effect profile and potential benefit warrant consideration of treatment.

References

1. Segers P, Speekenbrink RG, Ubbink DT, van Ogtrop ML, de Mol BA. Prevention of nosocomial infection in cardiac surgery by decontamination of the nasopharynx and oropharynx with chlorhexidine gluconate: A randomized controlled trial. *JAMA*. 2006;296: 2460–2466.
2. DeRiso AJ 2nd, Ladowski JS, Dillon TA, Justice JW, Peterson AC. Chlorhexidine gluconate 0.12% oral rinse reduces the incidence of total nosocomial respiratory infection and nonprophylactic systemic antibiotic use in patients undergoing heart surgery. Chest. 1996;109:1556–1561.Scheckler WE. Chlorhexidine gluconate for prevention of nosocomial infection in cardiac surgery. *JAMA*. 2007; 297; 1059–60.
3. Houston S, Hougland P, Anderson JJ, et al. Effectiveness of 0.12% chlorhexidine gluconate oral rinse in reducing prevalence of nosocomial pneumonia in patients undergoing heart surgery. *Am J Crit Care*. 2002;11:567–70.
4. Perl TM, Cullen JJ, Wenzel RP, et al. Intranasal mupirocin to prevent postoperative Staphylococcus aureus infections. *N Engl J Med*. 2002; 346:1871–1877.
5. Segers P, de Mol BA. Prevention of ventilator-associated pneumonia after cardiac surgery: prepare and defend! *Intensive Care Med*. 2009;35:1497–1499.
6. Scheckler WE. Chlorhexidine gluconate for prevention of nosocomial infection in cardiac surgery. *JAMA*. 2007; 297; 1059–60.
7. Klompas M, Speck K, Howell MD, Greene LR, Berenholtz SM. Reappraisal of routine oral care with chlorhexidine gluconate for patients receiving mechanical ventilation: systematic review and meta-analysis. *JAMA Intern Med*. 2014;174:751–761.
8. Hua F, Xie H, Worthington HV, Furness S, Zhang Q, Li C. Oral hygiene care for critically ill patients to prevent ventilator-associated pneumonia. *Cochrane Database Syst Rev*. 2016;10:CD008367.

47

An Intervention to Decrease Catheter-Related Bloodstream Infections in the ICU

The Keystone ICU Project

COURTNEY MAXEY-JONES AND EDWARD BITTNER

"We implemented a simple and inexpensive intervention to reduce [catheter-related bloodstream infections] in 103 ICUs. Coincident with the intervention, the median rate of infection decreased from 2.7 per 1000 catheter-days at baseline to 0 within the first 3 months after the implementation of the intervention."

—PRONOVOST ET AL.

Research Question: Can implementation of a bundle of involving five simple infection-control measures reduce catheter-related blood stream infections in the ICU?[1]

Sponsor: The US Agency for Healthcare Research and Quality

Year Study Began: 2003

Year Study Published: 2006

Study Location: 103 intensive care units in 67 Michigan hospitals

Who Was Studied: Patients from 103 intensive care units in 67 Michigan hospitals, representing 85% of all ICU beds in Michigan. ICUs included medical, surgical, cardiac, neurologic, surgical trauma units, and one pediatric unit.

Who Was Excluded: Data from 4 ICUs were excluded because these hospitals did not track the necessary data, and data from one ICU were merged and included with data from another ICU. In addition, 34 hospitals in Michigan chose not to participate in the project.

How Many Patients: A total of 375,757 catheter-days, which refers to the total number of days in which catheters were in place for all study patients. For example, a patient with a catheter in place for 7 days would represent 7 catheter days.

Study Overview: As part of the Michigan Keystone ICU project, participating ICUs implemented a series of patient-safety interventions including the use of a daily goals sheet to improve staff communication, a program to improve the culture of safety among staff, and an intervention to reduce the rate of catheter-related bloodstream infections. This analysis focuses on the intervention aimed at preventing catheter-related bloodstream infections.

Rates of bloodstream infections in participating ICUs were monitored for a three-month period prior to implementation of the safety initiative and for an 18-month period afterward.

Catheters were defined as those ending at or near the heart or in a great vessel close to heart (including peripherally inserted central catheters). Multiple lines within the same patient on the same day were counted as 1 catheter-day. CRBI were defined based on the National Nosocomial Infections Surveillance (NNIS) definition.

Study Intervention: In preparation for implementation of the safety initiative, each ICU designated at least one physician and one nurse as team leaders. Team leaders received training in the "science of safety" and on the components of the initiative. The team leaders, along with each hospital's infection-control staff, led implementation of the safety initiative at their respective institutions.

The safety initiative involved the promotion of five simple measures for preventing bloodstream infections:

- Hand washing
- Using sterile drapes during the insertion of central venous catheters
- Cleaning the skin with chlorhexidine disinfectant prior to catheter insertion

- Avoiding the femoral site for central line insertion whenever possible
- Removing unnecessary catheters

These practices were encouraged in the following ways:

- Clinicians received education about the harms of bloodstream infections and the importance of following infection control measures.
- A cart was created in each ICU with the necessary supplies for central line insertion.
- The central line carts included a checklist reminding staff to follow the preventive measures, and clinicians were instructed to complete the checklists whenever they placed central lines.
- During daily ICU rounds, teams discussed the removal of unnecessary catheters.
- Clinician teams received regular feedback on the rates of bloodstream infections among their patients.
- ICU staff were empowered to stop central line insertion if they observed that the preventive measures were not being followed (i.e., nurses and other staff had the authority to stop doctors who were not following the safety measures).

Follow-Up: Baseline rates of CRBI infection were obtained for ICUs not immediately implementing the intervention. ICUs were given a 3 month window to fully implement the intervention. Following the intervention, data was evaluated at 3 month intervals out to 18 months

Endpoints: Change in the rate of catheter-related bloodstream infections before and after the initiative began.

RESULTS

- The percentage of hospital ICUs stocking chlorhexidine in central line kits increased from 19% prior to the start of the initiative to 64% six weeks afterward.
- Mean infection rates decreased continuously throughout the study period, that is, the safety initiative became increasingly more effective throughout the study period (see Table 47.1).
- The safety initiative was effective among both teaching and nonteaching hospitals, as well as among both large (≥200 beds) and small (<200 beds) hospitals, though it appeared to be slightly more effective at small hospitals.

Table 47.1. KEY FINDINGS FROM THE KEYSTONE ICU PROJECT

Time	Median Infections Per 1000 Catheter Days at Study Hospitals[a]	Range of Infection Rates Per 1000 Catheter Days at Study Hospitals[b]	P Value for Comparison with Baseline Rates
Baseline	2.7	0.6–4.8	–
During Implementation	1.6	0.0–4.4	≤0.05
After Implementation			
0–3 months	0	0.0–3.0	≤0.002
16–18 months	0	0.0–2.4	≤0.002

[a] Catheter-days refer to the total number of days in which catheters were in place for all study patients. For example, a patient with a catheter in place for 7 days would represent 7 catheter days.

[b] The highest and lowest infection rates among study hospitals.

Criticisms and Limitations: Because there were no control ICUs that did not implement the safety initiative, it is not possible to prove that the initiative—rather than other factors—was responsible for the observed reduction in infections. The fact that infection rates didn't decrease substantially in other states during the same time period argues against an alternative explanation, however.

It is possible that the number of reported infections during the study period decreased simply because hospital staff changed the way that they diagnosed catheter-related bloodstream infections. For example, hospital staff may have underreported these infections during the study period simply because they knew that infection rates were being closely tracked. The authors believe this is unlikely, however, because "infection rates were collected and reported" according to prespecified criteria by "hospital infection-control practitioners who were independent of the ICU staff."

It is not known how well ICU staff followed each component of the initiative, nor is it known which component was most important for reducing infection rates. For example, it is possible that most of the observed benefit resulted from a single component of the initiative such as the use of chlorhexidine disinfectant.

Finally, it is not known how much time, effort, and cost each ICU had to invest to comply with the intervention. Resource utilization was likely modest, however, because the intervention was simple and did not require expensive equipment or supplies.

Other Relevant Studies and Information:

- A follow-up analysis showed that the reduction in catheter-related bloodstream infections in Michigan was sustained for an additional 18 months (total follow-up of 36 months).[2]
- A follow-up analysis also showed that implementation of the safety initiative was associated with a reduction in all-cause ICU mortality among Medicare patients in Michigan compared with the surrounding states.[3]
- A cost analysis examining data from six hospitals that were part of the Keystone ICU project suggested that the intervention saved money for the healthcare system: the average cost of the intervention was $3,375 per infection averted, however catheter-related blood steam infections typically cost approximately $12,000–$54,000 to treat.[4]
- The model used in the Keystone ICU initiative has been successfully implemented in other states including Rhode Island[5] and Hawaii.[6]
- Simple checklist protocols to reduce complication rates among surgical patients have also proven to be highly effective.[7,8]
- Studies have suggested that the rates of other hospital-acquired infections such ventilator-associated pneumonia can be greatly reduced with the use of simple checklist protocols.[9,10]
- Despite the successes of these safety initiatives, many hospitals in the United States and around the world do not consistently use these simple measures.
- A ten year analysis of the results of the Keystone Intensive Care Unit project demonstrated that reductions in central line-associated bloodstream infections were sustained through active involvement of hospital leaders, ongoing monitoring and feedback of performance.[11]

Summary and Implications: Implementation of a safety initiative involving five simple infection-control measures by ICU staff was associated with a substantial reduction in catheter-related bloodstream infections. While it is not certain that the safety initiative—rather than other factors—was responsible for the observed reduction, the study provides strong evidence that this safety initiative should be implemented widely.

CLINICAL CASE: REDUCING CATHETER-RELATED BLOODSTREAM INFECTIONS IN THE INTENSIVE CARE UNIT

Case History:
You are the Director of a 10 bed ICU in a small community hospital. Based on the results of this study, should you implement the intervention to decrease catheter-related bloodstream infections used in this study?

Suggested Answer:

This study suggests that implementation of a bundle consisting of five simple infection-control measures by ICU staff was associated with a substantial reduction in catheter-related bloodstream infections. The infection control bundle was effective in both large and small hospitals. However, implementation of a similar program at your hospital will require an investment of staff time and resources. In addition, the program may not work as effectively at your hospital as it did in the Michigan hospitals involved in this study.

As the ICU Director, you must decide whether the investment is worth it or whether the resources could be used in better ways (e.g., to hire more clinical staff). Many experts believe that implementation of the safety initiative used in this study would be a good investment, since the program is relatively inexpensive and seems to substantially reduce infections—which are not only harmful to patients but also expensive to treat.

References

1. Pronovost P, et al. An intervention to decrease catheter-related bloodstream infections in the ICU. *N Engl J Med.* 2006;355(26):2725–2732.
2. Pronovost PJ, et al. Sustaining reductions in catheter related bloodstream infections in Michigan intensive care units: observational study. *BMJ.* 2010;340:c309.
3. Lipitz-Snyderman A, et al. Impact of a statewide intensive care unit quality improvement initiative on hospital mortality and length of stay: retrospective comparative analysis. *BMJ.* 2011;342:d219.
4. Waters HR, et al. The business case for quality: economic analysis of the Michigan Keystone Patient Safety Program in ICUs. *Am J Med Qual.* 2011;26(5):333–339.
5. DePalo VA, et al. The Rhode Island ICU collaborative: a model for reducing central line-associated bloodstream infection and ventilator-associated pneumonia statewide. *Qual Saf Health Care.* 2010;19(6):555–561.
6. Lin DM, et al. Eradicating central line-associated bloodstream infections statewide: The Hawaii experience. *Am J Med Qual.* 2012;27(2):124–129. Epub 2011 Sep 14.
7. Haynes AB, et al. A surgical safety checklist to reduce morbidity and mortality in a global population. *N Engl J Med.* 2009;360:491–499.
8. de Vries EN, et al. Effect of a comprehensive surgical safety system on patient outcomes. *N Engl J Med.* 2010;363(20):1928–1937.
9. Bouadma L, et al. Long-term impact of a multifaceted prevention program on ventilator-associated pneumonia in a medical intensive care unit. *Clin Infect Dis.* 2010;51(10):1115.
10. Berenholtz SM et al. Collaborative cohort study of an intervention to reduce ventilator-associated pneumonia in the intensive care unit. *Infect Control Hosp Epidemiol.* 2011;32(4):305.
11. Pronovost PJ et al. Sustaining Reductions in Central Line-Associated Bloodstream Infections in Michigan Intensive Care Units: A 10-Year Analysis. *Am J Med Qual.* 2016;31(3):197–202.

Endocrine

48

The Normoglycemia in Intensive Care Evaluation

Survival Using Glucose Algorithm Regulation (NICE-SUGAR) Trial

DANIEL J. NIVEN AND HENRY T. STELFOX

"[Our] trial showed that a blood glucose target of less than 180 mg per deciliter resulted in lower mortality than a target of 81 to 108 mg per deciliter. On the basis of our results, we do not recommend the use of the lower target in critically ill adults."

—THE NICE-SUGAR STUDY INVESTIGATORS

Research Question: Can intensive glucose control (blood glucose target 81–108 mg/dl or 4.5–6.0 mmol/l) reduce 90-day mortality among adult patients admitted to medical and surgical intensive care units (ICUs)?[1]

Sponsor: Australian National Health and Medical Research Council, Health Research Council of New Zealand, Canadian Institutes for Health Research.

Year Study Began: 2004

Year Study Published: 2009

Study Location: ICUs in 42 hospitals in Australia, New Zealand, Canada, and the United States.

Who Was Studied: Adult patients (age ≥ 18 years) admitted to medical and surgical ICUs with a predicted ICU length-of-stay of at least 3 days, and an indwell-
ing arterial catheter.

Who Was Excluded: Patients were excluded if one or more of the following
were present:

- diabetic ketoacidosis or hyperosmolar state
- increased risk for hypoglycemia or a previous episode of hypoglycemia
  without full neurologic recovery
- predicted to be eating by second day in ICU
- admission to the ICU for ≥ 24 hours at the time of eligibility screening
- inability to obtain informed consent
- Death was predicted to be imminent

How Many Patients: 6,104

Study Overview: See Figure 48.1 for an overview of the study design.

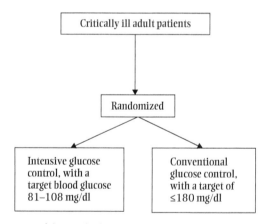

Figure 48.1 Summary of the study design.

Study Intervention: For both the intensive and conventional control groups,
glucose was managed with an insulin infusion titrated according to an algorithm.
The intervention was discontinued once the patient was eating or discharged
from ICU. For readmissions within 90 days of study enrolment, blood glucose
was managed according to original group assignments.

Follow-Up: 90 days

Endpoints: Primary effectiveness outcome: Mortality 90 days after randomization. Main safety outcome: Severe hypoglycemia (blood glucose ≤ 40 mg/dl or 2.2 mmol/l).

RESULTS

- 90 day mortality was increased in the intensive glucose control group compared with the conventional glucose control group
- Severe hypoglycemia (blood glucose level, ≤40 mg/dl) was more common in the intensive glucose control group compared with the conventional glucose control group.
- There were no significant differences between the two study groups in the mean ICU or hospital length of stay, duration of mechanical ventilation or need for renal-replacement therapy (Table 48.1).

Table 48.1. KEY FINDINGS FROM THE NICE-SUGAR STUDY

Outcome	Intensive Glucose Control	Conventional Glucose Control	Odds Ratio (95% CI)	P-value
Mean (standard deviation) time-weighted blood glucose, mg/dl	115 (18)	144 (23)	N/A	< 0.001
90-day mortality	27.5%[a]	24.9%	1.14 (1.02–1.28)[b]	0.02
Severe hypoglycemia, n (%)	6.8*	0.5%	14.7 (9.0–25.9)	< 0.001

[a] Among 3,054 and 3,050 patients randomized to intensive and conventional control groups, vital status at 90 days was available for 3,010 and 3,012 patients, respectively.
[b] Absolute mortality increase 2.6% (95% CI 0.4–4.8%); number needed to harm 38 (95% CI 21–250).

Criticisms and Limitations: The main limitation of NICE-SUGAR was its open label design: owing to the intervention, blinding clinicians to treatment assignment was not possible. Previous studies evaluating intensive glucose control were also open label.[2,3]

Significantly more patients in the intensive control group were treated with systemic corticosteroids (34.6% versus 31.7%, $p = 0.02$), although there was no significant interaction between receipt of corticosteroids and glucose control strategy.

The increased risk of severe hypoglycemia in the intensive glucose control group may be partially explained by the provision of intravenous insulin to patients receiving predominantly enteral nutrition at less than the recommended daily caloric intake. Previous trials examining intensive glucose control mandated the prescription of a minimal daily caloric intake mostly in the form of parenteral nutrition,[2,3] but reported similar incidences of hypoglycemia.[2,3] NICE-SUGAR employed a pragmatic approach to nutrition, and their results reflect a real world experience with intensive glucose control.

Other Relevant Studies and Information: Prior to NICE-SUGAR, other randomized trials evaluated the merits of intensive glucose control. The two most prominent studies originated from Leuven, Belgium.[2,3] In their first study (Leuven I), Van den Berghe and colleagues reported that providing intensive glucose control to predominantly surgical ICU patients decreased absolute mortality by 3.4%.[2] In their second study (Leuven II), the same authors reported no significant difference in mortality for patients admitted to a medical ICU.[3] Both studies reported an increased risk of severe hypoglycemia in patients treated with intensive glucose control compared to conventional glucose control (Leuven I, 5.1% vs. 0.8%; Leuven II 18.7% vs. 3.1%).[2,3] Three meta-analyses reported no significant differences in mortality, but increased risk of severe hypoglycemia for patients managed with intensive glucose control.[4-6]

In a follow-up study using their original clinical trial data, the NICE-SUGAR investigators found that moderate (blood glucose 41–70 mg/dl or 2.3–3.9 mmol/l) and severe hypoglycemia were associated with a significantly increased risk of death.[7] The incidence of hypoglycemia was highest among patients in the intensive control group. The risk of death was greatest among those who experienced severe hypoglycemia in the absence of insulin. These data suggest that glucose management strategies that reduce the risk of hypoglycemia should be the standard for critically ill adults.

Current guidelines suggest that a blood glucose ≥ 150mg/dl should trigger initiation of insulin therapy, titrated to keep blood glucose < 150mg/dl for most adult ICU patients and to maintain blood glucose values absolutely < 180 mg/dl using a protocol that achieves a low rate of hypoglycemia (blood glucose ≤ 70 mg/dl).[8]

Summary and Implications: NICE-SUGAR, a large, pragmatic clinical trial found that intensive blood glucose control increases the risk of severe hypoglycemia and mortality among adult patients admitted to medical and surgical ICUs. Conventional blood glucose control with a target of 180 mg/dl (10.0 mmol/l) or less should be the preferred approach in the management of critically ill adult medical-surgical patients.

CLINICAL CASE: GLUCOSE CONTROL IN THE INTENSIVE CARE UNIT

Case History:
You are the medical director for an intermediate volume ICU that admits adult patients with medical and surgical diagnoses. Based on the results of NICE-SUGAR, should your ICU adopt an intensive or conventional glucose control strategy?

Suggested Answer:
Following previous randomized trials of intensive glucose control, professional societies recommended intensive glucose control as standard practice for patients admitted to adult ICUs.[9] Subsequently, NICE-SUGAR demonstrated that intensive glucose control increases the risk of severe hypoglycemia and mortality, and should be avoided. Keeping in mind that hyperglycemia is also associated with increased morbidity and mortality, a conventional glucose control strategy wherein insulin is used to keep blood glucose less than 180 mg/dl (10.0 mmol/l) seems most appropriate.

Given the potential harms associated with an insulin infusion, conventional blood glucose control should follow a protocol that standardizes the frequency of blood glucose assessments and includes strategies to avoid hypoglycemia (e.g., minimum number of calories, mandatory dextrose infusion, etc.).

References

1. Finfer S, Chittock DR, Su SY, et al. Intensive versus conventional glucose control in critically ill patients. *N Engl J Med.* 2009; 360(13):1283–1297.
2. Van den Berghe G, Wouters P, Weekers F, et al. Intensive insulin therapy in critically ill patients. *N Engl J Med.* 2001; 345(19):1359–1367.
3. Van den Berghe G, Wilmer A, Hermans G, et al. Intensive insulin therapy in the medical ICU. *N Engl J Med.* 2006; 354(5):449–461.
4. Wiener RS, Wiener DC, Larson RJ. Benefits and risks of tight glucose control in critically ill adults: a meta-analysis. [Erratum appears in *JAMA.* 2009 Mar 4;301(9):936]. *JAMA.* 2008; 300(8):933–944.
5. Griesdale DE, de Souza RJ, van Dam RM, et al. Intensive insulin therapy and mortality among critically ill patients: a meta-analysis including NICE-SUGAR study data. *CMAJ.* 2009; 180(8):821–827.
6. Marik PE. Toward Understanding Tight Glycemic Control in the ICU. *Chest.* 2010;137(3):544.

7. Finfer S, Liu B, Chittock DR, et al. Hypoglycemia and risk of death in critically ill patients. *N Engl J Med.* 2012;367(12):1108–1118.
8. Jacobi J, Bircher N, Krinsley J, et al. Guidelines for the use of an insulin infusion for the management of hyperglycemia in critically ill patients. *Crit Care Med.* 2012;40(12):3251–3276.
9. Rodbard HW, Blonde L, Braithwaite SS, et al. American Association of Clinical Endocrinologists medical guidelines for clinical practice for the management of diabetes mellitus. *Endocr Pract.* 2007;13 Suppl 1:1–68.

49

Hydrocortisone Therapy for Patients with Septic Shock

The CORTICUS Trial

RYAN J. HORVATH AND EDWARD BITTNER

"Hydrocortisone did not improve survival or reversal of shock in patients with septic shock, either overall or in patients who did not have a response to corticotropin, although hydrocortisone hastened reversal of shock in patients in whom shock was reversed."

—SPRUNG CL ET AL.

Research Question: Among patients suffering from septic shock, does low dose hydrocortisone improve mortality?[1]

Funding: Supported by a contract from the European Commission, the European Society of Intensive Care Medicine, the European Critical Care Research Network, the International Sepsis Forum, and the Gorham Foundation.

Year Study Began: 2002

Year Published: 2008

Study Location: 52 Intensive Care Units (ICUs) in Europe and Israel

Who Was Studied: Patients who were 18 years of age or older hospitalized in participating ICUs with clinical evidence of infection, evidence of a systemic response to infection, and the onset of shock or organ dysfunction attributable to sepsis within the previous 72 hours.

Who Was Excluded: Patients not expected to live more than 24 hours, those on immunosuppression, those who were treated with long-term corticosteroids within the past 6 months or short-term corticosteroids within the past 4 weeks.

How Many Patients: 499

Study Overview: The Corticosteroid Therapy of Septic Shock (CORTICUS) study, was designed to evaluate the efficacy and safety of low-dose hydrocortisone therapy in a broad population of patients with septic shock (Figure 49.1).

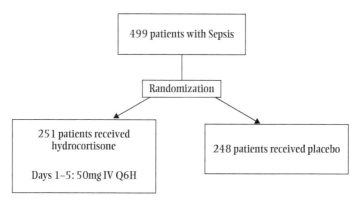

Figure 49.1 Summary of the study design.

Study Intervention: Patients in the treatment group received a 50 mg intravenous bolus every 6 hours for 5 days, then tapered to 50 mg intravenously every 12 hours for days 6 to 8, 50 mg every 24 hours for days 9 to 11, and then stopped. Vials containing placebo were identical to those containing hydrocortisone. All patients were also subjected to a short corticotropin stimulation test with blood samples taken immediately before and 60 min following IV injection of 250 mcg cosyntropin.

Follow-Up: 28 days, in the ICU, in the hospital and at 1 year.

Endpoints: Primary endpoint: Rate of death at 28 days in patients who did not have a response to corticotropin stimulation testing. Secondary endpoints: Rate of death at 28 days in patients who had a response to corticotropin stimulation testing, rate of death in the ICU, rate of death in the hospital, rate of death at 1 year, reversal of shock and length of stay in the ICU and hospital.

RESULTS

Primary Outcomes:
- There was no significant difference in the rate of death at 28 days among patients who did not have a response to corticotropin in the hydrocortisone group compared to the placebo group (39.2% vs. 36.1%, $p = 0.69$).

Secondary Outcomes:
- There was no significant difference between the rate of death at 28 days among patients who did have a response to corticotropin in the hydrocortisone group compared to the placebo group (28.8% vs. 28.7%).
- There were no significant differences between the rate of death in the ICU, hospital or at 1 year between the hydrocortisone and placebo groups.
- The duration of time until the reversal of shock was significantly shorter among patients receiving hydrocortisone for all patients ($P < 0.001$), for those who had a response to corticotropin ($P < 0.001$), and for those who did not have a response to corticotropin ($P = 0.06$).

Adverse Events:
- There was an increased rate of superinfection (relative risk 1.27, CI 0.96–1.68), new episodes of sepsis (relative risk 2.97, CI 0.61–14.59) or septic shock (relative risk 2.78, CI 1.02–7.58), hyperglycemia (relative risk 1.18, CI 1.07–1.31), and hypernatremia (relative risk 1.58, CI 1.13–2.22) in the hydrocortisone compared to the placebo group.

Limitations and Criticisms:
- Enrollment for this study was stopped at 500 patients instead of the planned 800 patients due to a combination of slow recruitment, expiration of study drug and termination of study funding. Due to lack of enrollment and decreased morality in the placebo group this study had power of less that 35% to detect a 20% reduction in the relative risk of death. Almost 25% of patients with culture-positive sepsis were determined not to have received appropriate antimicrobial therapy. The actual mortality rates among patients receiving appropriate antimicrobial therapy as compared with those receiving inappropriate antimicrobial therapy were not provided.

- The inclusion criteria of 72 hours for enrollment may have missed the optimal window of benefit for corticosteroid therapy.

Other Relevant Studies:

- The rationale for corticosteroid therapy for patients with septic shock originated from observations that patients with septic shock who had a reduced response to corticotropin were more likely to die and that the pressor response to norepinephrine may be improved by the administration of hydrocortisone. A prior randomized controlled trial by Annane et al.[2] suggested a survival benefit associated with the administration of hydrocortisone and fludrocortisone in patients with septic shock and relative adrenal insufficiency. As a result, corticosteroids became standard of care among such patients.
- Several differences between this and the prior study by Annane et al. may account for the differences in outcomes:
  - Patients in the Annane study, had higher severity of illness as indicated by SAPS II scores at baseline, and a much higher rate of death at 28 days in the placebo group (61%, as compared with 32% in the CORTICUS study). The lack of a treatment benefit in the CORTICUS study may be due to the enrollment of a population of patients with a lower mortality, for whom the risk of side effects of corticosteroid therapy outweighs its potential benefit.
  - Enrollment in the Annane study was allowed only within 8 hours after fulfilling entry criteria, as compared with a 72-hour window in CORTICUS.
  - Fludrocortisone was not administered to patients in CORTICUS as it was in Annane's study.
  - In the Annane study, corticosteroid treatment was stopped abruptly after 7 days, whereas in CORTICUS, therapy was tapered from day 5 to day 11. CORTICUS showed an increased incidence of superinfection, including new episodes of sepsis or septic shock, in the hydrocortisone group. This increased incidence of superinfection in the CORTICUS compared with the Annane trial may have negated the beneficial effects of corticosteroid treatment.
  - Care of patients with septic shock was markedly different in the two studies. The Surviving Sepsis Campaign guidelines were developed after the Annane study; their application could have resulted in the overall improved mortality rates observed in the CORTICUS study, reducing any additional benefit of corticosteroids.

- Meta-analyses that included both the CORTICUS and Annane studies found that the mortality benefit of low-dose hydrocortisone rose as the severity of illness increased. Prolonged (≥ 5 days) treatment with low-dose (≤ 300 mg/day) hydrocortisone was associated with reduced duration of vasopressor dependency in septic shock but was associated with increased risk of hyperglycemia, hypernatremia and possibly infection. Corticosteroid weaning provided no clear benefit over abrupt discontinuation.[3-5]
- The 2012 Surviving Sepsis Campaign guidelines recommend: "suggest against using IV hydrocortisone to treat septic shock patients if adequate fluid resuscitation and vasopressor therapy are able to restore hemodynamic stability. If this is not achievable, we suggest IV hydrocortisone at a dose of 200 mg per day."[6]

Summary and Implications: The CORTICUS trial failed to demonstrate a benefit on mortality with steroid therapy among patients with septic shock. Based on CORTICUS and other studies, the Surviving Sepsis Campaign guidelines no longer recommend steroids for all patients with septic shock. Corticosteroids should be considered, however, for patients with septic shock who do not respond to fluids and vasopressor therapy.

CLINICAL CASE: USE OF CORTICOSTEROIDS FOR THE TREATMENT OF SEPSIS

Case History:

A 68-year-old woman is admitted to the ICU with evidence of urosepsis including a white blood cell count of greater than 12,000, fever, and signs of early hypotension. Based on the CORTICUS Trial and related studies, would corticosteroid therapy be indicated in the following circumstances?

Scenario 1: The patient comes to the intensive care unit from the emergency department (ED) and after resuscitation with 2 liters of crystalloid fluid and appropriate antibiotic therapy she maintains a mean arterial pressure of greater than 65 mm Hg.

Suggested Answer:

Corticosteroid therapy would not be indicated as hemodynamic stability has been achieved with fluid resuscitation.

Scenario 2: Despite adequate fluid resuscitation and high dose vasopressor therapy the MAP remains less than 65 mm Hg.

Suggested Answer:
Given that this septic shock is refractory to both fluid resuscitation and vaso-pressor therapy, low dose corticosteroid therapy should be considered. Of note, corticosteroid therapy should be discontinued when the patient is no longer hypotensive.

References

1. Sprung CL, Annane D, Keh D, et al. Hydrocortisone therapy for patients with septic shock. *N Engl J Med.* 2008;358:111–124.
2. Annane D, Sebille V, Charpentier C, et al. Effect of treatment with low doses of hydro-cortisone and fludrocortisone on mortality in patients with septic shock. *JAMA.* 2002;288:862–871.
3. Sligl WI, Milner DA Jr, Sundar S, Mphatswe W, Majumdar SR. Safety and efficacy of corticosteroids for the treatment of septic shock: a systematic review and meta-analysis. *Clin Infect Dis.* 2009;49:93–101.
4. Moran JL, Graham PL, Rockliff S, Bersten AD. Updating the evidence for the role of corticosteroids in severe sepsis and septic shock: a Bayesian meta-analytic perspec-tive. *Crit Care.* 2010;14:R134.
5. Wang C, Sun J, Zheng J, et al. Low-dose hydrocortisone therapy attenuates septic shock in adult patients but does not reduce 28-day mortality: a meta-analysis of ran-domized controlled trials. *Anesth Analg.* 2014;118:346–357.
6. Rhodes A, Evans LE, Alhazzani W, et al. Surviving sepsis campaign: international guidelines for management of sepsis and septic shock: 2016. *Crit Care Med.* 2017 Mar;45(3):486–552

Musculoskeletal

50

Daily Interruption of Sedation with Physical and Occupational Therapy in Mechanically Ventilated Patients

MICHAEL WOLFE AND DANIEL SADDAWI-KONEFKA

"[D]aily interruption of sedation combined with physical and occupational therapy from the start of critical illness in patients on mechanical ventilation resulted in an improved return to . . . independent functional status . . . "

—SCHWEICKERT ET AL.

Research Question: In ICU patients receiving mechanical ventilation, does the early addition of physical and occupational therapy to daily interruption of sedation improve functional outcomes as compared to physical and occupational therapy at the discretion of the primary team?[1]

Funding: None

Year Study Began: 2005

Year Study Published: 2009

Study Location: University of Chicago Medical Center and University of Iowa Hospitals

Who Was Studied: Medical ICU patients, 18 years and older, who were mechanically ventilated less than 72 hours, expected to be on mechanical ventilation for at least an additional 24 hours, and meeting criteria for baseline functional independence (Barthel Index Score ≥ 70) prior to hospitalization.

Who Was Excluded: Patients with rapidly evolving neurological or neuromuscular disease, those intubated after cardiac arrest, those with irreversible conditions with >50% estimated 6-month mortality, those with raised intracranial pressure, those with multiple absent limbs, or those enrolled in another clinical trial.

How Many Patients: 104

Study Overview: See Figure 50.1 for an overview of the study design.

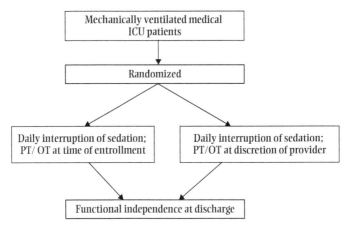

Figure 50.1 Design of a study by Schweickert et al.

Study Intervention: Patients were randomized to either daily interruptions of sedation combined with physical therapy and occupational therapy (intervention group) versus daily interruptions of sedation with physical and occupational therapy ordered at the discretion of the primary team (control group). Patients in either group who were medically unstable, or those whose goals of care were changed to comfort measures only, did not receive either the therapy or control intervention.

Unless contraindicated, all patients underwent a daily protocolized wean of sedation. When selected to receive therapy, physical and occupational therapists worked with patients during this interruption of sedation. Unresponsive patients received passive range of motion exercises of all limbs. With meaningful interaction, patients were progressed depending on their tolerance and stability, through active-assisted and active exercises in the supine position, to bed mobility activities, sitting balance activities, ADL and functional tasks oriented activities, and eventually transferring and walking. Therapy continued until discharge or return to baseline functional status was achieved.

Follow-Up: Hospital Discharge

Endpoints: Primary endpoint: The number of patients returning to independent functional status—defined as ability to perform six ADLs and independent walking—at time of hospital discharge. Secondary endpoints: Number of hospital days with delirium, number of days alive and breathing without assistance (ventilator-free days), and length of stay (ICU days and hospital days).

RESULTS

- Physical and occupational therapy occurred earlier in the intervention group than in the control group (median 1.5 days vs. 7.4 days from intubation, $p < 0.0001$). During mechanical ventilation physical and occupational therapy occurred for a median 0.32 hours per day compared with 0.0 hours per day in the control group. During the time not receiving mechanical ventilation, there was no difference in the duration of physical and occupational therapy (0.21 vs. 0.19 hours per day for study vs. control patients respectively, $p = 0.70$).
- In the intervention group, 59% of patients met criteria for independent functional status at time of discharge, compared with 35% of patients in the control group ($p = 0.02$).
- The intervention group had lower rates of ICU delirium (33% vs. 57% of time, $p = 0.02$) and hospital delirium (28% vs. 41% of days, $p = 0.01$) Amount of time spent in the ICU, total hospital days, and mortality did not differ between groups.
- Duration of mechanical ventilation was shorter in the intervention group. This was driven by a lower duration of mechanical ventilation

in non-survivors. Duration of mechanical ventilation for survivors was equivalent between groups.
• There was only one serious adverse event (desaturation < 80%) in 498 physical and occupational therapy sessions. Discontinuation of therapy as a result of patient instability occurred in 4% of all sessions, most commonly for perceived patient-ventilator asynchrony.

Criticisms and Limitations: This was a small study, involving only 104 patients. In addition the population was limited to medical ICU patients. This may limit its generalizability to other critically ill populations, including surgical and trauma patients, where physical and occupational therapy may be more challenging. Study enrollment was also limited to those who were functionally independent prior to admission, which may similarly limit external validity. Moreover, the unblinded nature of the trial introduces the possibility for unmeasured confounders.

Other Relevant Studies and Information:

• Several studies have demonstrated that early physical and occupational therapy can occur safely in the intensive care setting, including in mechanically ventilated patients.[2–5]
• A number of smaller studies support the results of this study, suggesting that early mobility in the intensive care population results in improvement of muscle strength, functional status, subjective feelings of wellness at time of hospital discharge, and possibly length of ICU and hospital stay (which was not demonstrated in this trial) (Table 50.1).[2,3,6–9]
• There is a paucity of other prospective, randomized trials analyzing effect of early mobility in mechanically ventilated patients.[10]
• Early mobilization is now recommended as a practice priority in adult intensive care units.[11,12]

Summary and Implications: Early physical and occupational therapy among ICU patients, including those who are mechanically ventilated, is safe and feasible. Early physical and occupational therapy during daily interruptions of sedation appears to improve functional status at time of discharge, and is associated with lower rates of both ICU and hospital delirium. Physical and occupational therapy should be considered early in a patient's ICU course.

Table 50.1. FINDINGS OF SIMILAR TRIALS

Study	Design	Intervention	Return to Functional Status	Ventilator Requirements	Delirium	ICU LOS (days)
Schweickert 2009	Prospective randomized controlled trial	Early PT/OT combined with sedation interruption	Functional independence in 59% study group vs. 35% control $p = 0.02$	Increased vent free days for study group $p = 0.05$	Decrease in study group 2.0 vs. 4.0 days $p = 0.02$	No difference 5.9 study vs. 7.9 control group $p = 0.08$
Morris 2008	Prospective cohort study	Implementation of mobility protocol in acute respiratory failure	—	No difference 7.9 days study vs. 9.0 days control group $p = 0.29$	—	No difference 7.6 study vs. 8.1 control group $p = 0.08$
Needham 2010	Prospective cohort study	QI project modifying sedation and physical therapy	Significantly higher rates of sitting, standing, transferring post-intervention; no difference in walking	—	Decreased post-intervention; 53% vs. 21% $p = 0.003$	Decreased 4.9 pre- vs. 7.0 post-intervention $p = 0.02$
Clark 2013	Retrospective cohort study	Implementation of early mobilization protocol	Discharged home: 67.9% post-protocol vs. 69.8% pre-protocol	No difference 7.8 days post-protocol vs. 8.9 days pre-protocol $p = 0.08$	—	No difference 10.4 post-protocol vs. 11.0 pre-protocol $p = 0.33$

CLINICAL CASE: DAILY INTERRUPTION OF SEDATION WITH EARLY PHYSICAL AND OCCUPATIONAL THERAPY IN A MECHANICALLY VENTILATED PATIENT

Case History:

A 71-year-old man with history of hypertension, hyperlipidemia, and past stroke with residual dysphasia but otherwise normal functional status is admitted to the medical ICU from home in respiratory distress. He is found to be febrile, tachycardic, and hypoxemic, with exam and imaging consistent with aspiration pneumonia. He is intubated for decompensated respiratory and mental status in the setting of his illness. Based on the findings of the Schweickert et al trial, what should be the approach to sedation and initiation of physical/occupational therapy in this patient to maximize likelihood of return to functional independence by hospital discharge?

Suggested Answer:

Based on the trial, this patient, who had normal functional status prior to his hospitalization, would benefit from daily interruptions of sedation and early initiation of physical and occupational therapy. Therapy should coincide with daily interruption of sedation. Under most circumstances, exercises are safe to perform and should begin even while mechanically ventilated. The patient's potential inability to actively participate in therapy should not preclude therapy. This practice of early therapy is associated with an increased rate of return to independent functional status at time of hospital discharge and lower rates of ICU and hospital delirium when compared to later initiation of therapy.

References

1. Schweickert W, et al. Early physical and occupational therapy in mechanically ventilated, critically ill patients: a randomised controlled trial. *Lancet.* 2009;373:1874–1882.
2. Burtin C, et al. Early exercise in critically ill patients enhances short-term functional recovery. *Crit Care Med.* 2009;37(9):2499–2505.
3. Morris P, et al. Early intensive care unit mobility therapy in the treatment of acute respiratory failure. *Crit Care Med.* 2008;36(8):2238–2243.
4. Pohlman M, et al. Feasibility of physical and occupational therapy beginning from initiation of mechanical ventilation. *Crit Care Med.* 2010;38(11):2089–2094.
5. Bailey P, et al. Early activity is feasible and safe in respiratory failure patients. *Crit Care Med.* 2007;35(1):139–45.

6. Chiang L, et al. Effects of physical training on functional status in patients with prolonged mechanical ventilation. *Phys Ther.* 2006;86(9):1271–1281.
7. Morris P, et al. Receiving early mobility during an intensive care unit admission is a predictor of improved outcomes in acute respiratory failure. *Am J Med Sci.* 2011;341(5):373–377.
8. Clarke D, et al. Effectiveness of an early mobilization protocol in a trauma and burns intensive care unit: a retrospective cohort study. *Phys Ther.* 2013:93(2):186–196.
9. Needham D, et al. Early physical medicine and rehabilitation for patients with acute respiratory failure: a quality improvement project. *Arch Phys Med Rehabil.* 2010;91(4):536–542.
10. Schaller S, et al. Early, goal-directed mobilisation in the surgical intensive care unit: a randomised controlled trial. *Lancet.* 2016;388(10052):1377–1388.
11. Calvo-Ayala E, Khan B, Farber M, Ely E, Boustani M. Interventions to improve the physical function of ICU survivors: a systematic review. *Chest.* 2013;144(5):1469–1480.
12. Hodgson C, Stiller K, Needham D, et al. Expert consensus and recommendations on safety criteria for active mobilization of mechanically ventilated critically ill adults. *Crit Care.* 2014;18(6):658.

INDEX